METHODS OF
DISGUISE
Second Edition

METHODS OF
DISGUISE
Second Edition

by John Sample

Loompanics Unlimited
Port Townsend, WA

Methods Of Disguise

Second Edition
© 1993 by John Sample

Published by:
Loompanics Unlimited
PO Box 1197
Port Townsend, WA 98368
Loompanics Unlimited is a division of Loompanics Enterprises, Inc.

Cover by Kevin Martin
Illustrations by Phoenix Ironworks.

ISBN 1-55950-096-4
Library of Congress Card Catalog 93-86361

Contents

INTRODUCTION

It's easy to define the word "disguise." Disguise is changing appearance to impede recognition or to fit into a role. Although this definition appears simple, it implies a lot. The main reason for disguise is its effect on others. This differentiates it from what's come to be called "body image" changing, in which dieting, plastic surgery, and other measures serve mainly for the effect on the self.

There are both legitimate and illegitimate reasons for assuming a disguise. Let's dispose of the illegitimate reasons first, because they're not the main concern of this book, although we will cover them for the sake of completeness.

The main reason for illegitimate disguise is to make an individual less recognizable by either law officers or witnesses to a crime. A bank robber may put on a stocking mask, hat, or sunglasses to confound witnesses. A fugitive from justice may try to change his appearance so that he no longer looks like the photo on the wanted poster.

The question inevitably arises whether a book detailing methods of disguise spreads knowledge which will mainly serve the criminal element, and therefore serves a negative social purpose. There are two good answers to this:

1. The criminal already knows the methods involved, having learned them from his criminal associates, cellmates in prison, or the copious crime shows on television. Hollywood movies spread the tradecraft of crime, not only showing the how-to, but explicitly portraying the scenarios in which criminal techniques are used. Newspapers often print accounts of crimes in very explicit detail, thereby informing all who can read exactly how criminals operate. Thus, the technical information is readily available to anyone who is interested.

2. Tools and techniques are not illegal and immoral in themselves. They can be well-used or misused. An automobile is not a criminal device, but a drunk driver or bank robber can misuse one. A camera is not a criminal instrument, yet it can serve for blackmail photos or pornography. A typewriter or word processor also isn't inherently a criminal tool, but a person can use one to write a ransom note, or to libel someone.

The situation is very much the same as the gun control issue. A firearm is not evil in itself, being useful for target shooting, hunting, plinking, and other legitimate purposes. However, individuals can and do misuse guns, either through carelessness or for criminal purposes. Tools and techniques are neutral: everything depends on the person using them.

This touches upon a basic problem in human history: New inventions can serve good or evil purposes. This theme runs through both history and fiction. Frankenstein's monster and other "mad scientist" stories are examples of perverted technology.

Let's now turn to legitimate uses of disguise, which happily outnumber the others.

Stage, screen, and television performers almost always use make-up, a moderate form of disguise, to obliterate wrinkles and other blemishes. Sometimes they change their appearances radically to play a role. An actor may play a person who is much older than he is, and the make-up artist must age him artificially. Sometimes men play women, and women play men, as in the film *Victor/Victoria,* another application of appearance-changing.

Prominent people sometimes wish to avoid recognition, perhaps because they fear kidnapping or assassination. More usually, they want to avoid the nuisance of autograph hunters, media reporters, and "paparazzi," photographers who prey upon the rich and famous and invade their privacy. Disguise for personal security is part of the technique of keeping a "low profile," essential for personal security. Often, it merely means avoiding being conspicuous, not putting on a false beard.

Police often use decoys in high-crime areas to lure muggers and arrest them in the act. This usually means that a police officer must assume the appearance and demeanor of a woman, old man, or even a drunk, to give the impression of vulnerability and encourage a prospective mugger to attack.

Disguise for the purpose of surveillance and shadowing is another need for both the police and for private investigators, and the individual following a suspect must periodically change his appearance so that the suspect does not notice the same profile behind him for a long period of time.

The 1971 Oscar-winning film *The French Connection* portrays a very realistic example of profile breaking during the chase scene in which "Popeye" Doyle, the police detective, follows his suspect from a restaurant, through the streets, and finally loses him in a subway station. During the pursuit, Popeye removes his hat, then his coat, to break his profile and avoid recognition.

A person who suspects that his or her spouse is adulterous may decide to follow him or her to check the real purpose of a trip. In this case, good disguise is essential, because it's critical to avoid recognition.

Runaways want to change their appearances. While the term "runaway" is usually applied to minors, an adult who has committed the same act is termed a "missing person." Running away from home is what we call a "status offense." It's illegal for a minor to do it, and the police can return him to his family. If an adult leaves home because he's unhappy with his situation, the police can't force him to return. In fact, many adults do run away each year, and this is illegitimate only if done to escape debt or child support.

The U. S. Marshal's Office of the Department of Justice has an official program to protect witnesses against retaliation from organized crime. The Federal Witness Protection Program relocates and provides new identities for such people. This program began in the 1960s and by 1976, over 2,000 people had received such aid. This program has been very successful, and by 1987, had relocated over 11,000 persons, including both witnesses and their families. By 1991, the total had increased to 12,982 persons.[1]

It's impossible to separate totally changes done for the effect on others from those done for the effect on the self. A person with a gross cosmetic defect, such as a harelip, will want to have this corrected, both for cosmetic effect and for the feeling of being "normal" that such correction will provide.

Physical defects, congenital or acquired, can be corrected by both surgical and non-surgical methods. A harelip must be corrected by surgery, but the fine scar that results can be covered by a mustache in a man. One well-known actor has done exactly that. Another man who had a port-wine stain on his face hid it with a beard.

Correction of a cosmetic defect can change the appearance so much as to make the person unrecognizable to someone who has not seen the individual since before the correction. In that sense, it's a disguise, as well as body-image work.

Reconstruction after injury is another reason for using methods of disguise. There may be prominent scarring, or a missing limb, and there are both surgical and non-surgical methods of concealing and correcting the defect. In fact, reconstructive surgery is a noted sub-specialty of plastic surgery, and the manufacture of prostheses serves to replace or conceal a missing part of the body, from a tooth to a limb. In some cases, the prosthesis is as good as the original, as in a tooth, and in other cases it's definitely limited, as with an artificial arm or leg.

Methods of disguise are extremely varied, as we shall see. They range from simple alterations in profile, such as putting on or removing clothing, to elaborate surgery.

What This Book Will Do For You

This book will provide an overview of disguise, how it works, and the reasons it works. We'll begin by studying how people see and recognize other people, and how to take advantage of failures in perception. We'll look at each class of disguise methods in detail, from superficial to surgical changes. We'll also study applications, such as stage and criminal disguises. From this book, you'll learn how to change your appearance, because we'll cover quick and temporary disguises, and permanent changes in appearance. You'll learn how to put together a pocket disguise kit, and more importantly, how to use it. The emphasis will be on practical, hands-on techniques.

There's been a lot of misinformation about appearance changing, much resulting from detective novels, whose authors would have you believe that a person's appearance can be changed radically, down to his fingerprints, by simple plastic surgery. We'll look at both fact and fiction, and present a realistic idea of what's possible, and how difficult and costly it is to attain.

This second edition contains new and updated information, as there have been developments in the field during the decade since *Methods of Disguise* first appeared. An appendix lists sources of supplies. Several new chapters provide details of new techniques for changing appearance and enhancing body image.

Notes

1. *Sourcebook of Criminal Justice Statistics,* 1991, Washington, DC, U.S. Department of Justice, Bureau of Justice Statistics, p. 67.

Chapter One

HOW PEOPLE IDENTIFY OTHER PEOPLE — LABORATORY RESEARCH

When considering methods of disguise, we have to understand how people recognize and identify other people. The police, of course, have studied this subject intensively over the years, because identification of perpetrators by witnesses is one of the ways in which they solve crimes. Police have learned a lot, empirically, about the ways in which people recognize other people. Surprisingly, this has seen confirmation for the most part by experiments under controlled conditions in psychological laboratories. What the police know by handed-down knowledge is, in fact, more accurate and comprehensive than the developments from laboratory research.

Laboratory research takes place isolated from real life, to separate the conditions being tested from extraneous factors. This is a valid way of proceeding, but what happens in the laboratory doesn't necessarily happen in real life. Out on the street, there are contaminating conditions which influence the results.

For example, in one series of studies all test subjects had normal eyesight, either with or without corrective lenses. In the real world, many people do not see well. Also in this series, the test subjects were all college students, presumably young and of better than average intelligence and education. On the street, we find people of all types and ages.[1]

Nevertheless, the available research is of value in giving us some scientific confirmation of what had previously been discovered by trial and error. It's unfortunate that the research isn't comprehensive enough to cover many real-life conditions.

One result of the laboratory tests was that the longer a subject studied a person, the more accurate subsequent recognition became. This unsurprising finding confirmed the common-sense knowledge that the better you know someone, the easier it becomes to pick him out in a crowd.[2]

Recognizing people from black-and-white or color photographs is a problem. Laboratory tests showed contradictory results.[3] One study showed that black-and-white mug shots were as good as color slides, while another showed that color improved the results. There were some differences in the way the tests were run, which probably accounts for the discrepancies. Common sense tells us that color provides another dimension, which should help recognition.

Discrepancies also have much to do with the way people perceive the world around them. Much research exists regarding the Rorschach, or ink-blot test, which was originally devised to diagnose mental abnormalities. Those who have worked with the Rorschach have found that normal people tend to identify objects by form more than by color, and that using color as the main means of identification is a sign of abnormality. Translated into real life, this means that we're likely to recognize a person by the shape of his facial features, color being secondary. Color is important, as many will describe the color of a person's hair and eyes when giving a description, but it's not the main determinant.

Memory generally decays with time, and the laboratory work confirms that the longer the interval between seeing the person to be identified and seeing the mug shots, the less accurate identification becomes.[4]

Race is important in recognition, and the effects of this are dominant in several ways. First, a person always notes another's race, because it's a feature easy to see and remember. On the street, witnesses usually state without hesitation the race of the person they describe, Some will even assign an ethnic group within a race to the subject they're describing, saying "looks Jewish," "Italian," etc.

Another effect of race is that people seem to be able to pick out individuals of their own race more easily than those of another race.[5] In the experiments, Caucasians were able to differentiate between subtleties of features of other Caucasians better than they were able to distinguish between Black subjects. This confirms what we often hear on the street: "They all look alike to me." One limitation of the research is that it covered only the responses of Caucasian test subjects, and there is no evidence regarding whether members of other races, such as Blacks or Asians, can differentiate well between individual Caucasians.

There was also an effort to determine which facial features were the most important in identification. Facial marks were most prominent. People also noticed ears, eye color, and teeth often.[6] The most important point which the study revealed was that people tend to notice more those features which stand out because they're uncommon, or different from the norm.[7] A scar, we know by experience, is easy to note and makes a person easy to identify later. We're also more likely to note a facial feature which, although normal, stands out because it's different from most, such as an unusually big nose, long hair, etc.

Skin color, as pertains to race, stood out as a main determinant.[8] Otherwise, complexion was not as important. Although this might seem an obvious point, its importance appears when we consider a police "line-up," the means by which a witness identifies a suspect. Most police officers know that a line-up must follow a certain format, as the identification may be invalidated in court if officers don't follow the format. For example, if the subject is Black, having him line up with six Caucasians is like dealing from a stacked deck, forcing his selection. Again, if the suspect is male, standing him up with several women will destroy the identification in court.

In a line-up, the police have each subject walk and speak, because they know from long experience that recognition is more positive if the witness observes the subject animate. They know that picking a suspect from a book of mug shots is often a frustrating process, as mug shots show only faces, and not how a person moves, walks, speaks, and all of the other subtle features that make up an individual. They use the mug book only to work towards narrowing the list of suspects, and the final identification must come by viewing the suspect in person. This is confirmed by an experiment in which the use of videotapes, color slides, and black-and-white photos were compared. The experimenters found that the extra dimensions provided by videotapes and color slides aided identification.[9]

The voice is very important, as it reveals speech patterns, accents, and sex. In one experiment, test subjects were able to identify the sex of the person by voice alone.[10]

As we've seen, laboratory research doesn't bring out any startling new discoveries, but confirms what we already know by intuition and experience.

Notes

1. Albert Zavala, Ph. D., and James J. Paley, *Personal Appearance Identification*, Springfield, IL: Charles C. Thomas, Publisher, 1972.
2. *Ibid.*, p. 25.
3. *Ibid.*, pp. 39, 298, 311-312.
4. *Ibid.*, p. 26, 312.
5. *Ibid.*, p. 41.
6. *Ibid.*, pp. 52-54.
7. *Ibid.*, p. 147.
8. *Ibid.*, p. 295.
9. *Ibid.*, pp. 311-312.
10. *Ibid.*, p. 298.

Chapter Two

HOW MUCH IS ENOUGH?

When considering disguise, we must look at the purpose for which we want it, balancing that against the cost and effort the disguise involves. There are basically two reasons for which you'd want to use disguise:

1. To make yourself less recognizable.
2. To impersonate someone else.

Changing appearance to impede recognition is by far the easier of the two. It doesn't matter if you end up resembling a particular individual, as long as you no longer appear to be you. This gives you considerable freedom in choosing a disguise. Your cosmetic changes could be as simple as growing a mustache or beard, or changing your clothing. A baseball cap and sunglasses, the favorites of armed robbers, also go a long way towards impeding recognition.

Impersonation, as we'll see, is far more complicated. You must change your appearance to resemble a specific person, and this entails more effort, explained more completely in the appendix on impersonation. It's most difficult when you try to impersonate a specific individual, rather than a member of a class. This difference is important in certain specific cases.

A police officer may make himself up to look like a derelict or senior citizen when assigned to a decoy operation. He need not resemble any particular person (muggers don't usually know their victims), but must hide the fact that he is a physically fit, armed, adult male.

Assuming the identity of a specific person, on the other hand, is very difficult, almost impossible in some cases, and utterly impossible in others. This is because the impersonator has to pass scrutiny by the impersonated person's relatives, friends, and acquaintances, and must mimic not only physical appearance, but also the speech, walk, and other behavior.

Whether this is possible, and whether it's economical to try, will be largely determined by the similarities in the two people. Obviously, it's impossible to disguise a 200 pound man to look like an 80 pound, 80 year old grandmother, even if the impersonator doesn't have to fool the family. If impersonator and subject begin with a close physical resemblance, it may be possible to disguise the impersonator to fool people at close range, although there will still be points of difference that a close investigation can reveal.

Generally, the less disguise, the better. A disguise can be so elaborate that it takes hours to assume, and the person cannot carry it well. An elaborate disguise is also easier to detect, especially if the intention is to impersonate a specific person. We'll see that trying to impersonate a specific person works only under specific conditions.

We'll begin with the simplest disguises and work up to the most complicated. We'll assess costs and benefits at each stage, giving you a framework on which to build a realistic evaluation of your needs and resources.

Chapter Three

A BASIC PHILOSOPHY OF DISGUISE

It's easy to understand that the simpler the disguise needed, the more effective it will be. We already know that the longer the person you're trying to fool scrutinizes you, the better his ability will be to recognize you later. It's also true that he'll have a longer opportunity to penetrate your disguise. Although the point of disguise is to change your appearance, you can use different approaches to this end. If you have a feature that makes you stand out from the crowd, you may be able to make yourself look more ordinary in many cases. If you already look fairly ordinary and forgettable, you can use a disguise that includes a striking facial feature, removing it when you revert to your original appearance.

There are obvious exceptions. If you're six feet, eight inches tall, you won't be able to reduce your height enough, even by stooping, to blend in with the crowd.

Using natural means of disguise is preferable because you need only what you already have at hand. A good example is the person who has worn a mustache for years. He can alter his appearance by shaving it off, and he can do this quickly. Growing a mustache takes much longer, but there's no danger of the adhesive loosening, as with a false mustache. Simply changing hair style, or clothing, can be very effective in some circumstances.

Other simple disguises use various make-up techniques and appliances. These may be cumbersome, and usually require buying devices and supplies, but have their uses. Many people wear eyeglasses, and these tend to stand out as identifiers. Changing to contact lenses is one way of suppressing this prominent feature.

We'll cover in detail the many techniques of disguise in the following chapters. Most are mechanical, but that should not obscure the fact that behavioral traits are an important part of the way people see you. You must be prepared to play the role totally if your disguise is to succeed. Professional actors understand this, and they spend more time learning to play a role than they do learning to apply make-up.

The disguise must fit the situation, and we'll look at various situations and examine what disguises are appropriate for them. Generally, the ideal disguise is one that you can create with minimal equipment and expense, and which goes on and off quickly. Unfortunately, few disguises fit this definition. Compromises are necessary, and judging the need for compromises and where to make them is the hardest part of assuming a disguise.

Chapter Four

NATURAL DISGUISES

It's common for people who want to change their appearance to change hair style, or in the case of men, to grow a mustache. It's less common for men to grow beards.

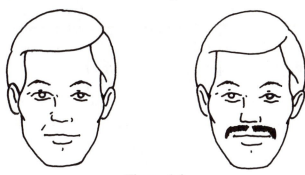

Figure 4-1

A mustache can alter the appearance and can be grown to hide a scar or a long upper lip.

One obvious use of facial hair is to cover what the wearer sees as a defect or weak point in the facial structure. A man with a very long upper lip may decide to fill the expanse with a neatly-trimmed mustache. A harelip repair scar is also easy to cover with a mustache. (See Figure 4-1.) Some of the men you see with beards are masking "weak" chins under the face fuzz. (See Figure 4-2.)

The effectiveness of hair in masking the features is beyond doubt. One of the annoying problems police face is that of the criminal who normally wears a large, scraggly mustache or beard during a crime, and then appears in court clean-shaven, confusing the witnesses.

One of the best aspects of facial hair is that the wearer can grow and shape it in many different styles, depending on the effect he wishes. A visit to a hair styling shop, or even an ordinary barbershop, will usually turn up a poster displaying different styles of mustaches. There's even more latitude with a beard. A beard can change facial contours, and mask the apparent shape of the head, which is an important feature in the system of identification by facial characteristics. A person with a thin face or pointed chin can grow his beard out to make his face appear fuller, or his chin bulkier. Likewise, a man with a receding chin can grow his beard out to an aggressive point, significantly changing his profile.

The main advantage of growing facial hair is that it's natural and, unlike false beards or mustaches, will not become unstuck at a critical moment. The main disadvantage is that it takes several weeks to grow and shape, which means that it doesn't work for quick-change disguise. On the other hand, it takes only minutes to shave one off, making a quick change possible in this direction. (See Figure 4-3.)

Changing hair style is an option open to both sexes, and many people change their hair styles during their lives for the sake of fashion, not disguise. (See Figure 4-4.) Scrutinizing the pages of fashion magazines shows many hair styles, for both men and women.

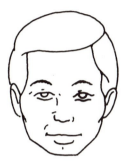 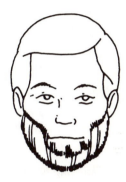

Figure 4-2

*A beard can change facial contours and disguise
the shape of the head. Growing a beard
will cover a weak chin.*

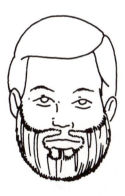 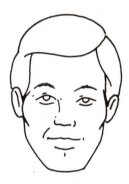

Figure 4-3

*Shaving facial hair takes only a few minutes
and can change the appearance radically.*

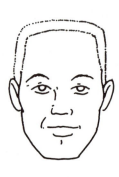 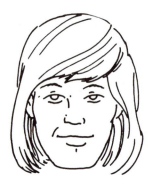

Figure 4-4

*Changing hair styles is an option open to both sexes,
and can serve for both disguise and fashion.*

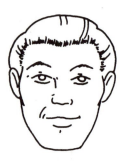 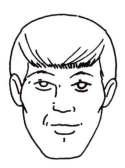

Figure 4-5

*Combing the hair forward can cover a receding hairline
and change the shape of the forehead.*

As with facial hair, growing the hair out takes a long time, perhaps too long for the purpose, although cutting it short takes only minutes. Restyling the hair takes a brush, comb, and a can of hair spray.

There are many ways hair can change appearance, modifying both the profile and full-face view. A person with a receding hairline can comb his hair high over the forehead to make it more prominent. (See Figure 4-5.) The apparent width of the forehead depends on how much hair covers it. The ears, which are also important in facial identification, can disappear under a mane of long hair. This is especially important if the person has prominent ears which attract attention. (See Figure 4-6.)

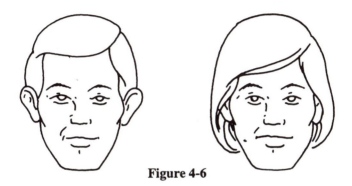

Figure 4-6

Growing the hair out covers protruding ears, thus hiding an important identification feature.

Long hair even has value in masking the wearer's sex. A man with delicate features and long hair can be mistaken for a woman, especially today, as both sexes wear similar items of clothing. While it's often true that body build and voice provide clues regarding sex, in many instances a witness may be unsure of the person's sex at first sight.

As with the hare-lip, mentioned above, hair is useful for covering facial deformities of various types. One man, born with a port-wine stain of the left side of his face, grew a beard to cover it. As facial deformities attract attention and are easy to remember, masking them is of great importance for disguise.

Although not a deformity, one of the most common easily remembered characteristics is baldness. Many men, as they age, tend to comb their remaining hair to cover a growing bald spot. If the baldness is slight, and the hair styling not too outlandish, few will notice the creeping baldness. However, we've all seen men with long strands of hair combed across the bald dome, from one side to the other, and this masking technique is so obvious that it makes the baldness more noticeable. (See Figure 4-7.)

Styling facial and head hair is more of an art than a science. Many people do it themselves with varying results. Probably the best way to begin is to have it done by a hair stylist, although the cost of professional hair styling is often ridiculously high, and then maintain the style, modifying it slightly when it becomes necessary.

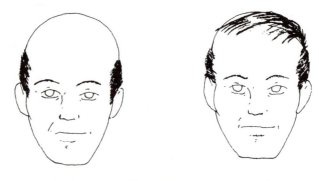

Figure 4-7

Baldness is easy to remember. A sloppy attempt to comb the hair over a bald dome can call attention to it.

A very effective method of changing appearance is available to people who are overweight: dieting. It usually works, but only if the dieter is serious, well-motivated, and persistent. It works slowly, taking from a few weeks to over a year depending on the weight loss desired and the dieter's ability to follow the regime firmly and avoid "cheating."

Loss of a lot of body weight always produces a significant change in appearance. (See Figure 4-8.) We've all seen before-and-after photos of people who have followed a certain diet plan in advertisements for them. Of course, these photos are those which show the most dramatic changes in a graphic manner. Most people won't show such great changes in appearance because they're not as grossly overweight as the people displayed in the ads. Still, most of us know people who have successfully followed diets and made significant changes in their appearances.

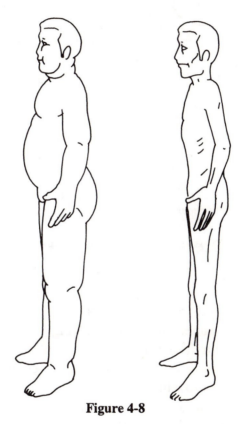

Figure 4-8

Weight loss or gain can dramatically alter the appearance.

Losing weight not only changes the body profile, but also results in remodeling of the face's contours. While the shape of the skull remains the same, and other features such as eyebrows and noses don't shrink, the cheeks and chin almost always recede with even slight weight loss. The cheekbones become more prominent as the mask of fat shrinks, and a double or triple chin slims to follow the throat's contours. (See Figure 4-9.)

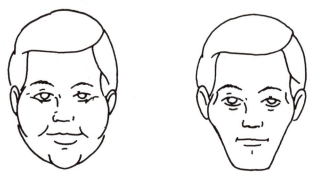

Figure 4-9

Weight loss affects the face as well as the body.
The cheeks and chin almost always shrink.

Diets: The Nitty-Gritty

Diet plans are among the most consistent selling self-help books, and this has been true for many years. New ones constantly appear, aimed at people seeking new answers to the same old problem. The reason for the continued large sales of diet books is simply that there are many people who read the books and don't follow them effectively.

The key to a successful diet is the willpower to persist. The authors of diet books emphasize various philosophies and schemes, not all of which are equally sound in scientific fact. Some place emphasis on reducing caloric intake. Others claim that calories themselves are not important, and only reducing the amount of carbohydrates ingested will work. Yet others insist that reducing food intake alone is not effective and that an exercise program is necessary, especially if they're selling exercise devices as a sideline. The time promised for effectiveness varies, with "crash" diets, "fourteen day" diets, and even indefinite promises such as "quick weight loss" diets.

It's remarkable that none of these work for everyone, yet they all work for someone. The experience of many people over many years has shown that the exact nature of the weight-loss program is not as important as the basic principle of reducing food intake consistently and persistently. Using drugs or fillers as appetite suppressants helps some people, but if they don't keep their food intakes down, they'll ultimately fail.

Dieting is aimed at a physical result, yet the psychological aspects are supremely important. Anyone starting on a diet should be sure that he wants to go through with it, and aware that any failure to restrict food intake will retard weight loss.

Motivation must be strong enough to overcome the temptations of over-eating. This is hard to do, especially if the dieter does not eat alone, but with friends and family, most of whom indulge themselves at the table. This leads to the temptation to follow the crowd and take an extra portion.

Any promise of a certain amount of weight loss in a certain period is valid only if a dieter doesn't cheat by punctuating his diet with periodic high-calorie meals. Promises of a given weight loss over time are, at best, generalizations that don't apply to everyone, because body builds, metabolisms, and body chemistries are different.

The other psychological factor affecting dieters is the mood swings that often accompany dieting. At first, the dieter notices several pounds of weight loss. Then a plateau comes, during which progress seems to stop. This is normal during dieting, as weight loss does not proceed along a fixed schedule, but follows an alternating pattern. The dieter will lose several pounds one week, then there will be a pause until weight loss resumes. During the pause, the dieter may become discouraged, and fall into a mental trough, unhappy at the lack of progress. He may become convinced that the diet doesn't work, or that he's gone as far as he can with that particular plan. If he then resumes eating at his old rate, he soon regains the pounds he's shed.

It takes confidence and mental stability to stick to a diet through both progress and plateaus. Avoiding discouragement is easier to say than to do, and many who start with serious resolve soon find their determination melting away while their fat doesn't.

Another problem is that dieting often fails in the long term. During the last few years, several long-term medical studies have shown that all diets have their failures, and that the usual result is weight loss in the short run, with a subsequent weight gain in the long run. Obviously, taking off weight is easier than keeping it off.

Just as a fat person can disguise himself by losing weight, a thin person can change his silhouette by gaining. In fact, if any person of "normal" weight were to gain or lose 50 pounds, his body and facial contours would change significantly. (See Figure 4-10.)

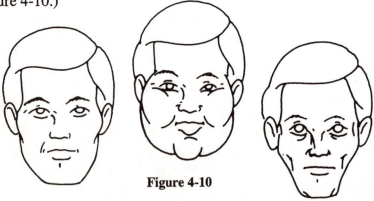

Figure 4-10

A weight gain or loss of fifty pounds will significantly alter the appearance. Here we see the effects on the face.

Chapter Five

MINOR AIDS IN DISGUISE

Many commonly available items serve well for disguising appearance. They work very well, are fairly inexpensive, and very cost-effective. Most of us already have some of them.

Clothing

A change of clothing will change appearance enough to be effective unless the person is already known to the subject. A pair of overalls can change the role the disguiser appears to be filling, as can a workman's cap or a hard hat. Any headgear masks the shape of the head. A brightly colored hat draws attention from the face, often being the feature remembered most clearly after the event. (See Figure 5-1.)

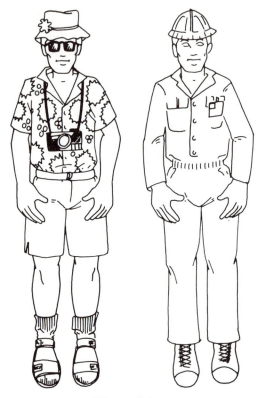

Figure 5-1

*Changing clothing makes a dramatic change in appearance,
as well as the apparent role the disguiser is filling.*

Eyeglasses

Experimental evidence has shown that wearing eyeglasses impedes recognition.[1] This experiment took place under laboratory conditions and did not accurately reflect real-life situations. In reality, the non-use of glasses has a greater effect than the experiment showed.

A person who normally wears glasses can impede recognition by removing them. If necessary, he can substitute contact lenses. Similarly, someone who does not wear glasses can put on a pair. (See Figure 5-2.) There are clear-lens eyeglasses available in some novelty stores, and some may choose this course. However, a simpler and cheaper way is to wear sunglasses, which mask the eyes and prevent a description of the shape and color of the eyes. Mirror sunglasses, which totally block a view of the eyes, are the most effective. (See Figure 5-3.) Persons who normally wear glasses can obtain prescription sunglasses.

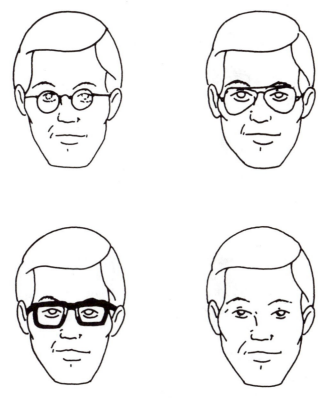

Figure 5-2

Putting on eyeglasses will impede identification. Someone who normally wears glasses can remove them or wear contact lenses to avoid recognition.

Contact lenses are a special case, for those who decide they want their special advantages. They can be ordered by mail[2] or purchased locally. They come clear or in colors, which is important for the person who wants to change the apparent color of his eyes. Someone with light-colored eyes can make his pupils appear darker, but it doesn't work the other way.

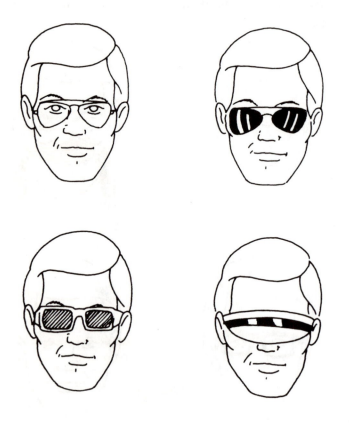

Figure 5-3

Sunglasses block a view of the eyes and are one of the most inexpensive and effective forms of disguise. They come in several varieties and styles, but mirror lenses are best for preventing later recognition.

Hair

Dyes and bleaches are inexpensive, and available in most department stores, supermarkets, and pharmacies, as well as beauty shops. Most are safe to use, but anyone using them should take care not to get any chemicals in the eyes as a matter of good general practice. Don't take for granted any claims of safety on the label.

In planning the use of dyes and bleaches, remember that most people see shapes more prominently than colors, and therefore use shape as a guide to recognition more than color. For best results, you should change your hair style, as well as color. (See Figure 5-4.)

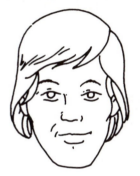 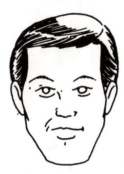

Figure 5-4

*Changing hair color is more effective
when the style is also changed.*

Props

Props are hand-carried items rather than apparel. A tool-box, for example, completes the picture suggested by overalls and a hard hat. A briefcase fits in with a three-piece suit. A shopping bag is doubly useful, because you can fold it up and put it in a pocket when not needed.

These props serve other purposes, especially as a way to carry other disguise items. Wigs, false mustaches, hats, etc., easily fit into these containers.

Disguise also serves another purpose beyond making the wearer less easy to recognize. If the purpose is surveillance, a prop such as a briefcase or tool-box can hold electronic devices for bugging, and the tools for installing them. (See Figure 5-5.) This is well-known to professionals in the field.

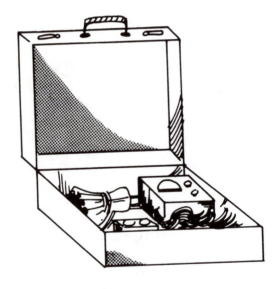

Figure 5-5

This attaché case is a convincing prop as well as a container for tools, surveillance devices, and quick-disguise items.

Notes

1. *Personal Appearance Identification,* p. 22.
2. Contact lenses of various types are available by mail from:
   Ideal Optics
   4000 Cumberland Parkway
   Atlanta, GA 30339
   Phone: (800) 554-7353
   Fax: (414) 434-8291
   Ideal Optics carries "Ciba Illusion" soft contact lenses, in various colors, which will change eye color. However, all contact lens orders have to go through an optometrist.

   International Contact Lens Laboratory
   63-52 Saunders Street
   Rego Park, NY 11374
   Phone: (800) 422-8489
   International provides contact lenses to change eye color, but they must be ordered through an optometrist.

Chapter Six

WIGS, MUSTACHES, AND OTHER FACIAL FUZZ

Wigs and false beards are the most popular items in the detective fiction writer's repertoire. Unlike plastic surgery, there's much factual basis for the fictional claims made for these items of disguise. A wig, mustache, or false beard can change a person's appearance radically, for relatively low cost, without the risks of plastic surgery, and with the option of instantly reversing the procedure.

As with other forms of make-up, the quality of the results depends very much on the care and skill of the user. He or she may buy a mail-order wig, slap it on, and with luck it will look natural. There are some problems, though, and those seeking effective disguises should be aware of them.

Generally, there are two types of hairpieces: full and partial. Costs run from ten dollars to over three hundred dollars, and they're available locally or by mail-order. Quality varies from excellent, natural-looking wigs to awful mops. The most important feature of a wig is its natural appearance, and this depends both on intrinsic quality and the care with which it's fitted.

A full wig that covers the top of the head doesn't have to be a perfect match, because it covers existing hair. A toupee, or partial hairpiece made to cover a bald spot, has to match existing hair. The wearer must also have it cut to fit so that it blends imperceptibly with existing hair. (See Figure 6-1.) It's possible for a very skilled wearer to do this himself. He must have the patience to cut a little at one time and try for fit, knowing that he can always remove a little more, but cannot put back what he's cut. For most people, the surest way is to buy a wig locally and have it professionally fitted. This one-time cost is worth it. Unlike natural hair, a wig doesn't need a haircut at regular intervals.

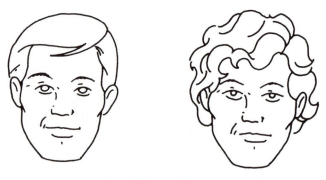

Figure 6-1

The wig is a popular disguise item. A full wig that covers the entire head doesn't have to match existing hair color or texture.

The main advantage of a wig over re-styling the hair is that it allows a quick appearance change. This isn't important to the person wearing a wig only for cosmetic reasons, but it can be important for disguise. As we've seen in previous pages, cutting the hair short is easy, but growing it back takes time.

The disadvantages of wigs are cost, delay in ordering and delivery, and possible discomfort, because some are uncomfortable to wear. This is especially true in hot climates; anyone living in this country's "Sun Belt" should consider comfort before obtaining a wig.

Buying a wig locally is easiest, and the staff helps the customer choose the wig, compare it to existing hair, and finally hand fit it to the head. One man, sensitive about his baldness, went to the extreme of going to his local beauty shop each morning to have his hairpiece fitted professionally, and combed to blend with his remaining hair. It cost a small daily fee for this service, but the result was excellent. The hairpiece was a perfect match, and undetectable even with close examination.

Anyone who wears a hat should note that a wig can slip or come off entirely. Even brushing the hand over the head can dislodge it, with potentially embarrassing results.

Mail-order Wigs

Buying a wig by mail takes longer, and there's always the possibility of dissatisfaction, because the buyer doesn't see the result until after he's paid for the wig and tried it for fit. Several companies sell wigs by mail, and some sell "as-is" while others offer money-back guarantees.[1]

There's quite a variety of hair products available by mail. (See Figure 6-2.) One company specializes in wigs and other hairpieces for Blacks.[2] For the do-it-yourselfer, there are excellent sections on false facial fuzz in several books on stage make-up.[3]

When ordering by mail, the customer has a choice of colors, hair styles, and synthetic or natural hair. For the best match, he should always send a sample of his hair with his order, although few companies suggest this in their catalogs. The choice between natural and synthetic hair is even more difficult, as hair varies in texture. Finding a match is usually a trial-and-error process, which is why sending a hair sample helps.

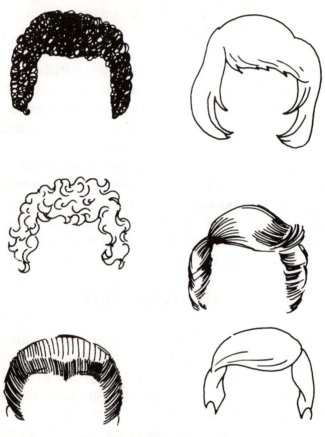

Figure 6-2

A great variety of wigs are available by mail.

Another point is important to the disguiser. Hair varies in color and texture in different light. An actor will choose a wig for one type of lighting, certain that it will look natural. Someone who wears a wig for disguise must take lighting into account, and understand that synthetic materials won't respond the same way to a change in spectral quality. Choosing natural hair is the safer course.

Applying A Wig

A full wig is usually designed with a net backing made of elastic and shaped to the head's contours. Applying the wig needn't be complicated. It can simply lie on the head, or the wearer may use an adhesive such as spirit gum to hold it in place.

Spirit gum is available in make-up supply houses and by mail,[4] and is especially made for prolonged contact with skin. This might appear a trivial point, but anyone planning to use adhesive on his skin should be aware that some can irritate. Others are toxic, and are not safe to use in contact with skin. This point may not be as important to the wearer of a wig as it is to someone planning to wear a mustache or beard. There's no adhesive made that is suitable for all people.

Some people have skin like armor plate, while others have very sensitive skin that becomes irritated by exposure to sunlight or detergents. Even medical adhesive tape, made for use on skin, is irritating to about twenty percent of the population, which is why we see "non-allergenic" tapes in pharmacies. Anyone using an adhesive should be especially careful when using it around the eyes, nose, and ears, as their delicate surfaces are more vulnerable to irritation.

To help match or blend wigs into existing hair, there are several easily applied hair colorings available from make-up supply houses.[5] These substances have a consistency between wax and Vaseline, and can be applied to lighten or darken hair. A commonly available item is mascara, for darkening eyelashes. Eyebrow pencils are obviously for eyebrows, although they can serve for other facial hairs in a pinch. Careful application will soften and blend in any line of demarcation between a wig and any fringe of hair showing from underneath. However, these are temporary make-ups, and come off with soap and water. Dyes and bleaches have longer lasting effects.

Assorted Facial Fuzz

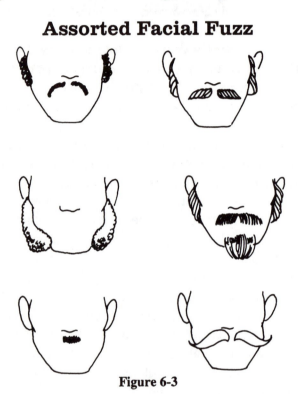

Figure 6-3

Sideburns and mustaches are available by mail or from local novelty shops. You can buy them pre-cut, or buy material and make your own.

Mustaches, beards, and sideburns are available pre-cut or, in some cases, the wearer can buy the material and make his own. (See Figure 6-3.) False eyelashes, usually made for women, are available in drug and department stores. Novelty shops sell other unusual disguise aids, and they're also available by mail.[6]

The type of material you choose depends on the effect you want. Mustaches and beards are available in many styles, from the toothbrush "Hitler" mustache to the full facial hair of the rugged outdoorsman. However, for those who want to make their own, there's crepe material available in bulk. You can cut this in various shapes and style it for the desired effect. Crepe material is kinky and if you want straight strands, you must straighten it with a steam iron before shaping.

Crepe is also suited to wispy mustaches and sideburns, not strongly shaped ones with sharp lines. Crepe will do for someone who wants to look like an old man with scraggly whiskers, or for a Santa Claus, but not for a relatively young man with a neatly-trimmed mustache. (See Figure 6-4.)

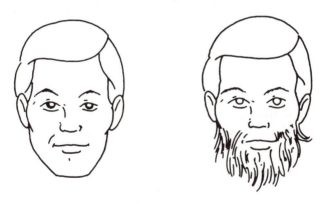

Figure 6-4

*Crepe serves to make wispy whiskers but is unsuitable
for tight, neatly trimmed mustaches or beards.*

Note that crepe has other disadvantages. Application is a long and tedious process, which involves painting the face with spirit gum and applying the crepe a few strands at a time. For repeated use, you should apply it to a latex base on your face, so that you can peel it off in one piece. However, this may simply be too much trouble.

Another disadvantage is that you must color the crepe to the suitable shade for you, using make-up cosmetics, an additional step. The skill needed to apply crepe is more than most of us want to take time to develop. This is good reason to consider ready-made face fuzz.

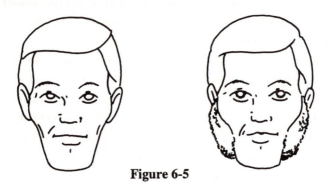

Figure 6-5

Sideburns fill out a thin face.

Ready-made mustaches are by far the most convenient to use. Color match is not as important as with wigs, because facial hair often is a different shade than hair on the head. Texture is not as critical, except that mustaches tend to have straight, not kinky, hairs. Sideburns are often kinky, and must blend in with the scalp hair where they meet.

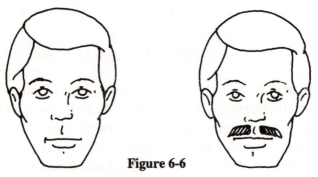

Figure 6-6

A *mustache fills in the gap between nose and mouth.*

The effect of a mustache or set of sideburns is the same whether the facial hair is natural or artificial. Sideburns fill out a thin face (see Figure 6-5), and a mustache can break up the space on a long upper lip (see Figure 6-6) or, in the case of a bushy mustache, partly or totally hide the lips.

False eyebrows are less effective and don't see much use except by actors making up for a role. Modifying the appearance of the eyes by donning eyeglasses is far easier than using eyebrow prostheses. False eyelashes are mainly used by women, as a beauty aid. Like eyebrows, their effectiveness in disguise is minimal.

One commonly available aid to keeping a false beard, sideburns, or wig in shape is hair spray. Without it, applying the hairpiece will always require careful combing to make it look right. Some prefer to spray and shape the hairpiece while wearing it, and this is often the most convenient way to do it, as we're accustomed to combing or brushing our hair normally. In other cases, a person will prefer to use a wig block, a plastic device shaped like a human head.

In principle, spraying any facial hair is time consuming. Some users of disguise, however, may have to apply hairpieces quickly. Applying adhesive with a brush, waiting for it to dry, and then cementing the hairpiece in place takes too long. In such instances, using double-faced tape may solve the problem, although it can't give as good a result as careful hand-fitting with conventional methods.

There are several brands and types of double-faced tape, some with adhesive on a foam plastic base, others using cellophane or mylar, and at least one type which is just a band of adhesive. This is 3M's Scotch brand #665, which comes in a roll that sells for about three or four dollars, and consists of a layer of adhesive on a paper support. The paper isn't part of the tape, and its use is to keep the layers of adhesive separate on the roll. In use, it's necessary to tear off a suitable length and apply it sticky-side down to the skin or hairpiece, peeling off the paper backing afterwards. The adhesive layer is very thin, and once the paper is removed, easily shaped to fit.

In use, you carry the mustache with the adhesive on and the paper separator in place until you're ready to use it. You then peel off the paper, and the facial fuzz is easy to apply quickly.

As with other tapes and adhesives, double-faced tape may irritate some people's skin. Generally, the longer it remains in contact with skin, the greater the chance of adverse effects.

Notes

1. Wigs are available by mail from:

Bob Ellis
280 Driggs Avenue
Brooklyn, NY 11222
Phone: (718) 383-3379

Franklin Fashions Corp.
103 East Hawthorne Avenue
Valley Stream, NY 11582
Phone: (800) 621-5199

Jack Stein Make-up Center
80 Boylston Street
Boston, MA 02118
Phone: (617) 542-7865

Bob Kelly Cosmetics, Inc.
151 West 46th Street
New York, NY 10036
Phone: (212) 245-2237

2. Wigs styled for Blacks are available from:

Afro World Hair Co.
7276 Natural Bridge
St. Louis, MO 63121
Phone: (800) 325-8067

3. *Stage Make-up*, by Richard Corson, 6th Edition, Engle-wood Cliffs, NJ, Prentice-Hall, Inc., pp. 208-249.
4. Spirit gum is available from Bob Kelly Cosmetics, address above, and other stage make-up suppliers.
5. Hair whitener is available from Bob Kelly Cosmetics, and comes in a half-ounce tube. This is one of the easiest to apply disguise products.
6. Mail-order beards, mustaches, sideburns, etc., are available from Bob Kelly Cosmetics, and Jack Stein. Additional sources of supplies are in the *Sources* appendix.

Chapter Seven

CRIMINAL DISGUISES

A quick study of disguises often used by criminals will help round out the role of disguise in modern life. Criminal disguises often differ from what we normally call "disguises" because they're not intended to help the wearer play a role, but only to impede later recognition. In some cases, criminal disguises don't help the criminal blend into a situation, but are very conspicuous. A ski mask, for example, worn by a bank robber certainly makes him stand out in a crowd, but it serves the purpose by totally obscuring his face.

"Street-wise" criminals become fairly sophisticated after some experience, aided by coaching from other criminals, and they learn the basics of identification procedures and the rules of evidence. Successful criminals are also very practical, and they keep their disguise methods as simple as they can, because excessively elaborate methods are difficult and time-consuming.

A simple and effective disguise for an armed robber, for example, is a ski mask and a "211" jacket.[1] (See Figure 7-1.) The robber carries his ski mask wadded in a pocket, donning it at the last moment and removing it when it's safe. An alternative is the nylon stocking, which distorts the features and compresses into even less space than the ski mask. However, these are less comfortable than ski masks, and for some the nylon catches their eyelashes and feels awkward.

A total face covering solves many problems, hiding facial contours, blemishes and scars, and it frustrates security measures such as cameras. Knowledgeable criminals understand that sometimes this is not enough, because witnesses can identify robbers by other features, such as the color of the hands, speech patterns, accents, and gait.

A disadvantage of the ski mask or nylon stocking mask is that the robber must don it immediately before the act, risking that witnesses may see him unmasked. In some types of businesses, such as convenience stores,[2] cameras cover the entire premises. Some, such as the "Crime-Eye," use hidden cameras that begin snapping a series of still pictures when a clerk presses a hidden button. Others, such as closed-circuit TV cameras, are overt and run continuously, and sometimes record the perpetrators unaware before the start of the robbery.

CCTV cameras are visible, and some are designed to be conspicuous because they have a red light at the front. Some "cameras" are actually dummies, low-cost enclosures designed to resemble CCTV cameras, used as deterrents. Perpetrators who "case" the premises while planning the crime realize that they have to don masks before coming into the camera's view.

Surprisingly, there are few attempts to destroy the cameras. Anyone planning a robbery must contend with at least two possibilities, first that before he can destroy the camera, it will have photographed him onto videotape and that the recorder is at a remote location, and that while he's destroying one, there may be others recording him, some of which may be hidden.

Judging the best moment to remove a mask is also a problem, for anyone trying to escape into a crowd with a mask will be conspicuous. Witnesses will be able to provide descriptions of the perpetrator's face if he unmasks.

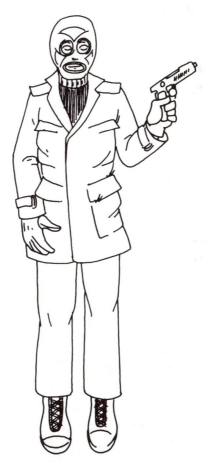

Figure 7-1

A ski mask and "211" jacket comprise a simple disguise
often used in armed robberies.

The advantage of the nylon stocking mask is that it's easy to dispose of it inconspicuously after the need for it is over. A nylon stocking discarded on a sidewalk won't attract any attention.[3] Another advantage is that nylon mesh fabric does not retain fingerprints.

More sophisticated criminals use other disguises that appear natural, so that they can walk the streets without attracting undue attention. An effective disguise is inconspicuous, yet covers or changes the face enough to impede recognition.

False mustaches, beards, and sideburns are effective because they don't have to pass close scrutiny and they hide part of the face or change its contours. A cap or sweater in a loud color aids the effect, drawing attention from the face. Eyeglasses and sunglasses, especially the mirror kind, are among the best and most easily available disguises.[4]

Wigs, cheap and easy to don when used simply to hide the real hair, are very useful to a criminal. A cheap, poorly-fitting wig doesn't look natural, but prevents witnesses from seeing the suspect's real hair.

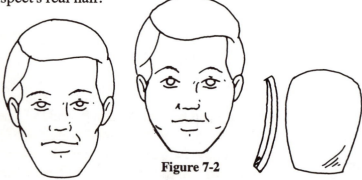

Figure 7-2

Mouth inserts change the shape of the face and modify the voice. Front and side views of one type of insert are shown at right.

Criminals also use mouth inserts. These can be cotton, plastic, rubber, or even wadded newspaper. They swell the cheek contours and if placed under the palate, even change the pitch of the voice. (See Figure 7-2.)

For those with dental plates, removing them changes the lips and jaw line. A spare set of dental plates, with one or more teeth blacked out or missing, will provide the illusion of missing teeth, an attention-capturing feature that obscures the description. (See Figure 7-3.)

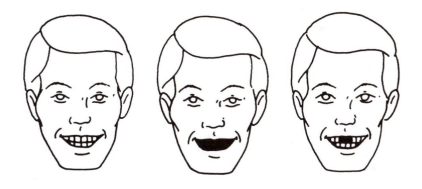

Figure 7-3

*For those who wear false teeth, a spare set of dental plates
can be altered to show missing teeth.*

Nostril inserts, made of cork, rubber, or plastic, widen the nose while allowing the user to breathe almost normally. These are tubes shaped to fit inside each nostril. (See Figure 7-4.) One use of nostril inserts is to allow a Caucasian suspect to resemble another racial type. Make-up darkens the skin, but his Caucasian facial bone structure will give him away. Widening the nostrils helps complete the illusion.

Body shape and contours are another way suspects change their appearance. Padded clothing can make the wearer seem to be dozens of pounds heavier. (See Figure 7-5.)

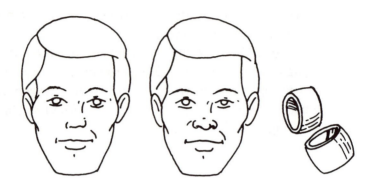

Figure 7-4

*Nostril inserts widen the nose, yet allow normal breathing.
Inserts are shown on right.*

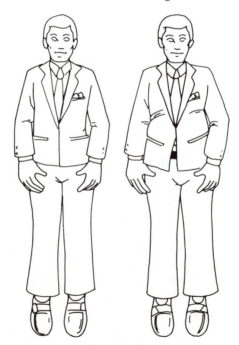

Figure 7-5

Padded clothing adds dozens of pounds to the apparent weight.

While casing the premises, the prospective armed robber may notice that there are inconspicuous height indicators within the cameras' fields of view. Rulers are often painted on the doors, because suspects must enter and leave through them, giving witnesses the opportunity to estimate their heights fairly accurately. A subtle height indicator is a patterned wallpaper; comparison of the pattern with the suspect's figure in photographs allows estimating his height precisely.

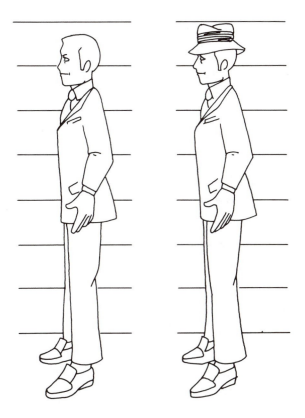

Figure 7-6

A hat conceals the hair and adds to the apparent height.

Countermeasures include wearing a hat to make the precise height hard to measure, as well as to conceal the hair. (See Figure 7-6.) Another technique is wearing "lifts." (See Figure 7-7.) These are shoes with built-in "elevator" inserts, or after-market inserts which he can put into his shoes to make him look taller. Some cowboy boots have high heels which add two or three inches to the height.[5]

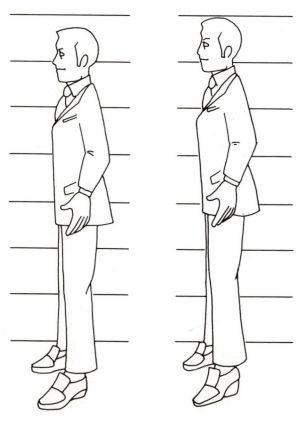

Figure 7-7

Shoe lifts add inches to apparent height, and are seldom detectable in photos taken by security cameras. Witnesses often don't scrutinize the suspect's feet, either.

Falsifying distinctive markings is another way to impede identification. Tattoos are extremely easy to fake, and almost every child knows that an indelible pencil will, when dipped in water, mark the skin in a shade that resembles tattoo ink. Fake tattoos, also obtainable on tracing paper, are easy to apply and remove with soap and water. A tattoo on the face makes an excellent back-up to a face mask or stocking, in case a bystander sees the mask being donned or removed.

Temporary tattoos are commercially available, and offer more elaborate designs than possible with home-made applications. These are brilliant-color plastic film tattoos mounted on paper backing, and they apply with water. When fresh, they look much too bright for a real tattoo, and it's necessary to tone them down with baby powder or even make-up powder.[6]

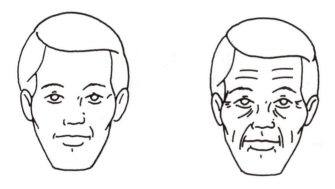

Figure 7-8

Aging lines are effective and easy to apply.

The more ambitious suspect with a flair for artistry can simulate scars. There are many ways to put fake scars on the face with stage make-up.[7] It's easy to fake scars using rough and ready materials bought in a pharmacy.[8]

Simulating warts and moles with mascara is another way of creating facial blemishes. Rouge simulates a port-wine stain.

The suspect willing to take more time with his disguise can draw in age lines with make-up or mascara pencil. This technique is simple, and requires only filling in normal lines in the skin to make them appear thicker and deeper. This requires little practice to learn, and can quickly add years to the apparent age. (See Figure 7-8.)

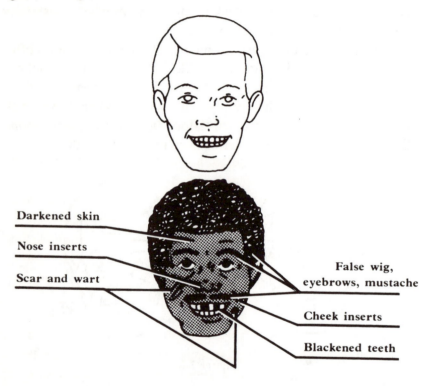

Darkened skin

Nose inserts

Scar and wart

False wig,
eyebrows, mustache

Cheek inserts

Blackened teeth

Figure 7-9

*A complete transformation! With the proper materials
and careful application, a young Caucasian could pass
for an older Black person, as long as
close inspection isn't possible.*

Gloves have always been important to the criminal, and today are absolutely essential. Traditionally, gloves have covered defects in the hands, as well as hand skin color for those wishing to pass as members of another race. Missing fingers, tattoos, and other blemishes are conspicuous recognition marks.

Fingerprints are far more important today than ten years ago, because of the introduction of Automated Fingerprint Identification Systems, or AFIS. Previously, it was necessary for a technician to make manual comparisons of suspect fingerprints at a crime scene. This was time-consuming, and normal practice was to compare the suspect print with those of a short list of possible perpetrators. Today, computerized AFIS systems allow comparing a single fingerprint against millions of others contained in the computerized database. The computer run required to identify the California "Night Stalker" killer, for example, took only 90 minutes.

Criminal disguises today are easier to use than ever, and a wider variety is available to the lawbreaker. However, the criminal must pay closer attention to detail, because some crime detection methods have improved drastically.

Notes

1. "211" jacket is a term used by police on the West Coast to denote a leather or vinyl jacket, long enough to cover below the waist and conceal a pistol tucked into the pants. It's loose, masking the contours of the handgun, and the pockets are large enough to carry a ski mask and the proceeds from the robbery.
2. These are victims of robberies so often that in some parts of the country they're called "Stop N' Robs."
3. *Disguise Techniques,* Edmond A. MacInaugh, Boulder, CO, Paladin Press, 1984, p. 28.

4. Several types of mirror sunglasses are available by mail-order from:

Johnson Smith Company
4514 19th Street Court East
PO Box 25500
Bradenton, FL 34206-5500
Phone: (813) 747-2356
Fax: (813) 746-7896

5. Lifts and elevator shoes are not criminal devices, as they're made for those who want to appear taller for esthetic reasons. They are limited because most add only about two inches, except for boots, to apparent height. They're locally available, and some companies sell them by mail-order:

Richlee Shoe Company
PO Box 3566
Frederick, MD 21701
Phone: (800) 343-3810
(301) 663-5111

Richlee's catalog shows elevator shoes of various styles, including what they call "sport shoes" that resemble sneakers. Dress and casual shoes add about 2" to height, while cowboy and work boots provide about a 3" increase. However, footwear styles are for men only.

Inner Lifts Footwear Co.
2205 Oxford Road
Raleigh, NC 27608

This company sells only lifts. These are inner soles and heels to fit inside the shoe, but prices are in the $20 range.

Lifts are adaptable to most shoe styles, but are limited by the space inside the shoe.

6. One supplier is:

Don Ling's Removable Tattoos and Fantoos
PO Box 309
Butterfield, MN 56120
Phone: (800) 247-6817
(507) 956-2024
Fax: (507) 956-2060

7. *Stage Make-up*, Richard Corson. This book provides many ways to modify facial features for the stage. Many methods described are too cumbersome for use on the street, but Chapter 13 explains making and using fake scars.
8. *Armed Robbery,* by Carl Dorski, Fort Pierce, FL, Roadrunner Publications, 1978, pp. 7-10. This is a how-to book covering various aspects of planning and carrying out armed robberies. The section on disguises, while short, is full of precise information.

Chapter Eight

MAKE-UP

Make-up is what first comes to mind when thinking about disguises. As with other aspects of disguise, reality conflicts with the popular image. While donning make-up can make a sharp and dramatic change in appearance, results are usually less spectacular. Nevertheless, while make-up isn't as effective as other means of hiding the features, it's worth a look.

There are two roughly overlapping categories of make-up: ordinary cosmetic make-up and stage make-up. The first is for people who just want to enhance their looks by putting red into their cheeks or covering rough skin and other small defects. Stage make-up is more elaborate, and is for use on stage, and in front of film and TV cameras.

Stage Make-up

Everyday make-up is readily available and easy to use. Stage make-up has always been a special case. It came about centuries ago, when actors needed to modify their appearances to play their roles. At first, it was crude paint or creme, roughly applied, to change skin color. It was often obviously unrealistic, and even today this is true of some types of make-up, such as clown colors. Often, make-up is accompanied by a prosthesis, such as a wig or false nose, and the effect and realism depends on the skill of the person applying the make-up.

During the last century, the use of calcium carbide lamps, "limelights," was common for indoor stage illumination. These produced bright, harsh, greenish-white light which gave a bleached appearance to the actors' complexions. Using dark skin cream became necessary to avoid a stark, ghost-like appearance. Thus make-up became a standard tool for all stage performers, not only those playing a role requiring a change of appearance.

Electric lights changed this somewhat, as the rosy glow of incandescent bulbs did not bleach the complexion the way greenish-white carbide lamps did. Another type of stage light which came into use was carbon-arc, with its intense ultra-violet emissions, and actors still needed make-up. The movie industry, at the outset equipped only with monochromatic films which inaccurately reproduced the natural colors in shades of black and white, became another large user of stage make-up. An important factor was that the films of those days, with their deficient color rendition, were also very insensitive, with single- or double-digit speed ratings instead of the three-digit figures we take for granted. During the early days a film speed of 100 was science fiction, and insensitive films needed high light levels to record at the short shutter speeds of cinematic photography.

The story was much the same when television came into use. Unlike the sensitive hand-held videocam used to make the "Rodney King" videotape using street lights, early kinescope cameras needed high light levels to pick up images. Early TV was black-and-white, and the rendition of skin color in gray tones was poor. Color TV did not see widespread use until the 1960s.

Today, with color media common in both the film and TV industries, and with quartz-iodide lamps replacing arc and carbide lights on stage, skin tones appear more natural. However, actors still use make-up to enhance their appearance. Today, the emphasis is on subtlety, especially because today's much improved cameras can record every flaw.

Medical Make-up

There's a sub-category of make-up which falls across the other two. We can call this "medical make-up," which began as make-up prescribed by doctors to cover various skin conditions. Acne cream is one common type.

What makes these creams and lotions different from other make-up is that they contain some sort of "medication," usually non-prescription, for a skin ailment. Apart from this, medical make-up is thicker and heavier than typical "pancake" make-up material.[1]

Street Make-up

Ordinary street make-up is very familiar, and everyone has seen displays of creams, lipsticks, and various types of eye shadow and mascara which fill the cosmetics departments of almost every store in the country. They enhance the beauty of the user's features, and modify or conceal both real and imaginary defects in the complexion. Advertisements tell us that dry skin is undesirable, and that there are preparations to correct this. Oily skin is also a fault, according to cosmetic manufacturers, and they make cosmetics for that as well.

The basic make-up is the "foundation": a creamy, flesh-colored preparation that hides small blemishes and serves as a sort of primer coat for other make-up. Foundation comes in many tints, to match every complexion. Consistencies vary from thick liquid to creams. All do two things: cover and color. Some people are convinced that they look unnatural and unhealthy because they're too pale, and they choose a foundation that is darker than their skin color.

Some preparations darken the skin by producing a tan. These stimulate pigmentation, and one well-known lotion brand is "Coppertone,"[2] available in Walgreen's and other drug stores. Another widely-advertised brand is "Bain de Soleil."[3] Walgreen's also markets its private brands, including tanning oil and lotion, and tan amplifier, all available in Walgreen's stores.

Protective lotions, such as sun blocks, are quite different. These are ultraviolet light barriers which limit penetration of ultraviolet light, the wavelength which causes both tanning and sunburn. Some, however, contain a tanning ingredient, making the distinction less clear.

Another type of suntan product merely simulates a tan, and is known under the generic term "bronzing powder." "Brush A Tan" is one brand.[4]

"Pancake" make-up is heavier than a foundation, and is for covering more noticeable blemishes. A heavy enough pancake fills in wrinkles, covers liver spots, and masks other aging marks. A special make-up, "Covermark," available in some local pharmacies, is for covering port-wine stains and scars.

Eye shadows and mascara accentuate the eyes, as do false eyelashes. Lipstick will change the color of the lips, but this is not really a disguise.

With street make-up, the most important point is subtlety. Carelessly applied or excessive make-up will be conspicuous, and the best effect comes from applying make-up with a light touch, unlike stage make-up. Street make-up must withstand close examination for a long time, and defects in application will become obvious.

Major cosmetics manufacturers put out small make-up kits for accentuating highlights and shadows in the face. These are comparable to stage make-up, but again cannot count as disguises because they don't change facial contours.

Removing Wrinkles

Heavy face make-up, such as foundations and cremes, fill in wrinkle lines. These are strictly make-ups, and rub off easily. However, it's now possible to obtain a longer-lasting effect.

During the middle 1980s, doctors and their patients discovered a side-effect of high-potency vitamin-A creme normally used to treat acne: it suppresses wrinkles. The effect varied with different people, and was not permanent, but certainly lasted far longer than blemish cremes. Vitamin-A creme works by first making the skin tissue swell, then peel. Dead and wrinkled skin layers slough off, revealing the fresh layer of skin underneath.

One type of Vitamin-A creme is "Retin-A," available only by prescription. It's fairly expensive, at about $20 for a half-ounce tube, but a little bit goes a long way. A non-prescription brand is "Retinol."[5] None of these products erase wrinkles permanently. Still, a temporary effect is more desirable than using make-up.

Darkening Hair Quickly

There are hair dyes that darken hair with successive applications, and others that require ammonia or peroxide. A quick

way is to use Bigen permanent powder hair color to cover gray
hair, enhance or darken natural hair color, and to restore hair
color faded by sun or sea. Use by mixing the powder with
water, according to instructions, and applying the mixture to
the hair with a brush. You leave it on until the hair becomes the
shade you want, usually between 20 and 30 minutes, then rinse
the mixture out of your hair and shampoo.[6]

Tooth Whitening

Removing heavy stains from the teeth impedes recognition.
There are several stain removing toothpastes available in pharmacies, and one from a California company sold in make-up
supply outlets. This is EpiSmile.[7] The effects are not immediate, taking about three weeks to appear. Brushing twice daily
with EpiSmile gradually lightens tobacco and other stains, although it's not effective against antibiotic stains.

Disguise Make-up

Make-up for disguise has three purposes:
1. To suppress identifying scars and blemishes.
2. To change facial features.
3. To create false blemishes to mislead witnesses.

Generally, the more ambitious the purpose, the more time
and skill it takes to apply the make-up. Stage make-up is very
comprehensive, and some of it is unnecessary on the street.
Street use imposes no need to compensate for harsh lighting,
and some techniques require more skill than most of us have.

Anyone with enough experience in stage make-up can write
his own shopping list, but the rest of us are better off starting
with a kit. Kits contain more than just the basics, and this allows some experimentation. One suitable kit is Bob Kelly's
Creme Stick Make-up Kit. [8] This contains:

Six full-size creme sticks
Eight creme liners
Liquid latex
Make-up pencils
Brushes
Hair whitener
Molding putty
Translucent powder in a shaker
Powder puff
Black stipple sponges
Applicator sponge
This kit comes in a small cardboard box, along with an instruction leaflet.

Make-up Techniques

It's important to stress that not all stage make-up techniques are suitable for the street. Let's cover the more practical ones:

Covering Scars and Blemishes

Scars, acne, and other blemishes, if they're not deep pits, will respond to creme make-up. (See Figure 8-1.) Choose a shade closest to your skin tone and apply it with the fingers, blending it into the skin at the edges of the area you're covering. Cover the creme with a light coat of neutral face powder. If you have deep pits, you can fill them with molding putty, but with many pits this becomes time-consuming.

You can simply apply molding putty with the fingers, but it requires a special technique. Molding putty is a soft, tacky, and waxy compound, made to stick to the skin. When handling it, you should apply a coat of vegetable jelly, such as K-Y, to your fingers, to keep the putty from sticking to them. Apply the putty on clean skin, before using any creme or foundation, because these will keep the putty from adhering to your skin. Be sure to "feather" the edges so that there is no clear line where the putty begins. Feathering means working the putty into a very thin coat at the edges, so that it blends imperceptibly into the texture of your skin. Cover the putty with creme stick, to blend the color in with the surrounding skin.

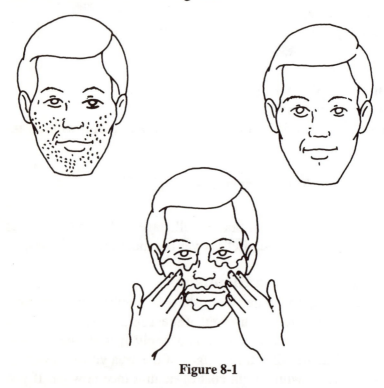

Figure 8-1

Scars and acne can be covered by applying creme make-up, blending it in with the fingertips, then coating with powder.

Use liquid latex, available from several sources, to fill in small scars and pits. You apply this in thin layers with a brush, letting each layer dry before applying the next. However, latex is white, not flesh-colored like molding putty, and covering it with creme is essential. Again, a light coat of powder will make it look more natural.

If a heavy coat of make-up is necessary, stippling with a coarse sponge, such as those included in make-up kits, will help produce a texture like that of skin. Stippling is a technique that requires practice, not just rough knowledge. Reading about it will explain the technique, but only actual practice will teach you how to do it.

Fake Bump on the Nose

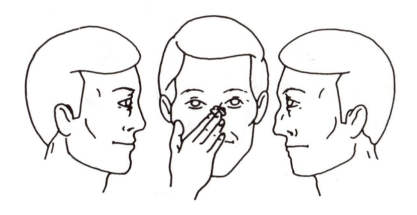

Figure 8-2

The profile can be changed by building up a lump on the nose with molding putty and covering it with make-up.

This is easy to apply with molding putty, but the fake bump tends to fall off, especially if you wear glasses and the bridge rests on the edge of the artificial bump. To apply, wet your fingers with K-Y, break off a suitable lump of molding putty, and apply it to the spot on your nose you've chosen to build up. Use care in shaping, and blend the bump in with the contours of your nose. In blending, work from the inside out, using light pressure at first, then more as your fingers travel towards the outside. It's important to make the outside edge as thin as possible, feathering it to blend into your skin without leaving a line. The flesh-colored putty may match your skin closely. If it doesn't, apply creme and blend it in, then finish the job with a light coat of powder. (See Figure 8-2.)

Aging the Face

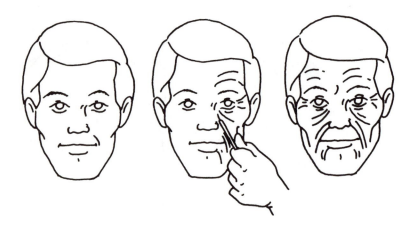

Figure 8-3

Create aging lines by darkening existing wrinkles
on your face and blending them in slightly.

In many ways, this is the easiest make-up to apply because you don't have to re-shape your face, and the materials are easy to use. The basic technique is to enhance the wrinkles already on your face. In front of a mirror, make a face to show the wrinkles, and apply liner with a pencil at the bottom of each wrinkle to make it appear deeper. An alternative technique is to use a fine brush to apply creme of a deeper shade than your skin tone. There are several ways to darken the bottom groove of a wrinkle, and they all work if you use them carefully so as not to make it obvious that you're wearing make-up. The trick is to blend the make-up in, so that the lines don't stand out by being too sharp. (See Figure 8-3.)

Using these techniques is almost as easy as reading about them, but don't expect too much. Making a twenty-year-old over to look like eighty takes much more than this.

Some highlighting on top of the forehead will help the illusion. Use a creme slightly lighter than your skin tone. If necessary, you can blend two shades in the palm of your hand to get the right tone before applying. A white creme stick, as found in the Bob Kelly kit, will lighten any shade with which you blend it.

Hair whitener will make the hair seem either gray or white, depending on the original color and how much you use. Hair whitener comes in stick form, and is easy to apply, as long as you remember to blend it in with the fingertips after stroking it onto the hair. A small amount at the temples will suggest a "distinguished" look, but if you prefer, you can whiten your whole head of hair. If you wear a mustache, a good effect is to whiten the mustache and leave the hair natural, or vice versa. The contrast will draw attention away from the rest of your face.

As this make-up is designed to fool people up close, it's vital to avoid a sloppy job. Good make-up of this sort has to be subtle, blending in with your natural face, not clashing with it. It's also important to remember that making up the face is not all that it takes to simulate age. Someone with an aged face and unlined, youthful hands will be obvious even to many unobservant people.

Another point is that there's more to the impression of age than a few wrinkles. Gait and mannerisms also help to create an impression of age. A person with a lined face and a light, springy step will not look natural. It's vital to be able to play the role.

Creating Scars and Defects

There are several materials useful for creating scars and other defects, and the result depends heavily on the skill and imagination of the user. One technique is to build up a scar line using latex or putty, and to fill it in with ruddy cake make-up. (See Figure 8-4.) Skillful blending and a light touch are essential. A variation on this theme is to build up a ridge and then slice it down the middle with a butter knife, filling in the bottom with dark make-up. A drop or two of artificial blood can make the scar seem like an open wound.

Bob Kelly sells "Scar Material," designed for application with a brush. Applying this in the desired shape, thin layer on top of thin layer, will build up a scar effect. To blend it in with surrounding skin, apply a coat of base make-up over it. Bob Kelly also provides a make-up trauma kit for simulating various injuries and scars.

At this point, it's worth repeating that these make-up materials can cause adverse effects in people who have sensitive skin. Although designed to be non-toxic, some of the other materials and chemicals used in conjunction, such as the acetone necessary to remove the scar material, are definitely toxic. It's worthwhile to apply a small amount of the substance on the forearm, or another area of the body away from the face, to test the skin for sensitivity.

It's also possible to use a prepared artificial scar, applying it when needed with spirit gum or other adhesive. This is a useful technique at times because it allows you to make the scar when you have the time to do it, saving it for later use. You have the time to make it exactly right, or to revise it if it's not right the first time.

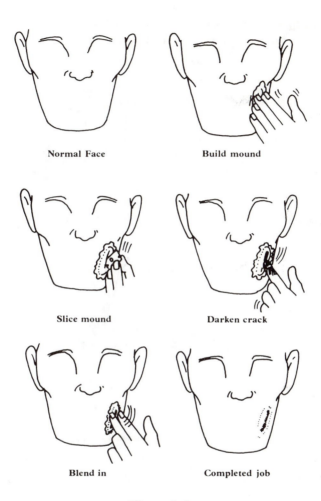

Normal Face

Build mound

Slice mound

Darken crack

Blend in

Completed job

Figure 8-4

*You create a scar line by using liquid latex or putty, ruddy make-up
for the scar, and regular make-up to blend it in.These drawings
show the technique using putty, which is faster. Liquid latex
requires application with a brush, layer on top of layer,
to obtain the right thickness.*

Applying a previously prepared scar to the face also requires care to blend it in, usually the application of a light coat

of liquid latex with a sponge to give it texture, then a thin layer of powder, with a final coat of creme if necessary to match the tone and texture of your skin.

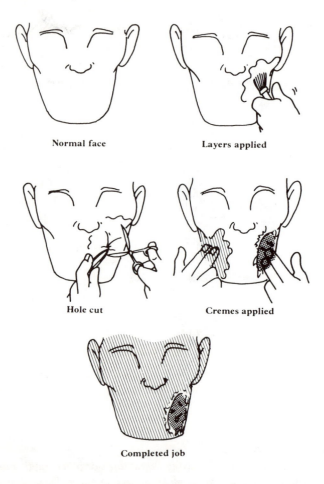

Normal face   Layers applied

Hole cut   Cremes applied

Completed job

Figure 8-5

Red face creme in conjunction with liquid latex simulates a severe sunburn. The edges of the latex patch simulate peeling, and darker creme in the center creates the fresh skin uncovered by the peeling.

These steps are what make applying make-up more of an art than a science. You cannot depend strictly on a formula, but have to do the job "by eye," because everybody's skin is different.

Simulating a severe sunburn is more involved, although it's the same basic process. The first step is to apply two very thin and even coats of latex to the area, letting each layer dry thoroughly before applying the next. Another layer or two will probably be necessary for best results. This is something you have to judge when applying the material, adapting the technique to your own skin.

While waiting for each layer to dry, try not to move the skin, as this can cause wrinkles. After the last layer dries, apply a layer of powder, then a light coat of sunburn shade creme. Then use a tweezer to pick up a corner of the latex patch and lift it away from the skin. Use scissors to cut out the center of this section. The edges should peel back and simulate the skin peel that comes after sunburn. Then apply some creme in the hole, selecting a slightly redder shade. This will simulate the fresh skin that is uncovered by a sunburn peel. (See Figure 8-5.)

You may want to create a reusable scar or defect for repeated applications. This requires a casting that you can build up to produce a final product colored to match your skin tone. We'll cover this more thoroughly in the chapter on castings.

Missing Tooth

This technique is probably the easiest of all, and only requires black-out tooth wax. A child's non-toxic black wax crayon makes a good substitute. (See Figure 8-6.) First, clean the teeth with a paper towel, to remove both tartar and moisture that would impede adhesion of the wax. Next, apply the wax. The limitation of this technique is that it's crude, and the make-up will be visible to anyone who takes a close look. It works best if you normally keep your lips together, so that anyone observing you will see the "gap" only during the fleeting moments when you open your mouth to speak. However, if your normal expression is to keep your lips spread slightly, this method won't work well.

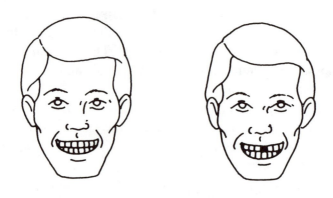

Figure 8-6

A missing tooth effect is created with black-out tooth wax or child's non-toxic wax crayon.

Learning to Use Make-up

One good text on stage make-up is *Stage Make-up*, by Richard Corson, listed in the *For Further Reading* section. There are several others, most of which are well-illustrated as is essential with how-to books of this sort.

Additional information on use and techniques is available from suppliers of stage make-up, many of which provide instruction leaflets with their products. These are brief, no-nonsense instructions that outline the techniques step by step. Most are freebies supplied with catalogs. Others come with the products themselves.

For the serious student, it's worthwhile to study these texts carefully, not only to gain information about specific products and techniques, but to learn the limits of the materials available. Some techniques, such as the temporary face-lift, can simulate the results of plastic surgery for a short while, but are very cumbersome to apply and require more skill than a particular individual might be willing to develop.

Limitations of Make-up

Unfortunately, disguise consists of much more than a superficial change in appearance, and the exact depth of the transformation required depends on the situation. We've already noted that for some changes, such as aging, cosmetic work is not enough, and there must be a corresponding effort to act the role.

Another point is that make-up isn't permanent, and this has its positive and negative aspects. In most instances, an irreversible change would be undesirable. Make-up is also very vulnerable to damage. Skin preparations rub off easily, and simply wiping your hand across your face, or scratching an itch, can damage the make-up and instantly destroy the illusion.

In one sense, this can be an advantage, as it makes make-up fairly easy to remove for a quick change. Actually, reverting to the original appearance takes less time than the original change, because most make-up wipes off with cold cream.

Applying make-up takes time, which varies with the effect you want and your skill. This points up the need to practice and develop your skill. Reading a chapter in a book won't make you an expert, and you must practice to sharpen your skills. This can take many, many hours.

Using make-up to play a role over a prolonged period is very difficult, because it's necessary to touch up and even renew the make-up repeatedly. Even a semi-permanent make-up such as hair dye or bleach requires frequent touch-ups as your hair grows out, to avoid showing the original color at the roots of your hair.

Nevertheless, there are many uses for make-up, for someone who understands its limitations and is willing to undertake efforts to develop the skill. With proper selection and application, make-up works well in limited circumstances.

Notes

1. Cabot Laboratories, of Central Islip, New York, 11722, has a brand called "Clear Perfection," which includes corrective cover creme, corrective finishing powder, corrective retouch concealer, and leg & body cover creme.
2. Coppertone is manufactured by Schering-Plough, Memphis, TN 38151.
3. This is manufactured by Proctor & Gamble, P.O. Box 599 Cincinnati, OH 45201. Phone: (800) 283-4879.
4. This is manufactured by Glamazone Cosmetics, Lakewood, NJ 08701, and is available in pharmacies such as Walgreen's.
5. Retinol was available at the time of writing for $5.00 plus $2.00 shipping & handling from:

Beauty Solutions
334 East Lake Rd., Suite 171
Palm Harbor, FL 34685

6. Bigen is available from:

Nishimoto Trading Company
2747 S. Maly Avenue
Los Angeles, CA 90040
Phone: (800) 835-8844

Sig Frends Beauty Supply
5270 Laurel Canyon Blvd.
North Hollywood, CA 91607
Phone: (213) 877-4828
(818) 769-3834

7. Available from:

   EPI Products
   PO Box 2975
   Beverly Hills, CA 90213
   Phone: (800) 444-5347

8. Bob Kelly Cosmetics, Inc.
   151 West 46th Street
   New York, NY 10036
   Phone: (212) 819-0030
   Kelly carries a variety of make-up products made for use on stage, screen, and television. See the list of sources at the end of the book.

Chapter Nine

CASTING PROSTHESES

Traditionally, the way to produce special effects, such as bumps, scars, jug ears, etc., has been to build them up on the subject with wax or clay while applying make-up. While some special effects are removable and reusable, in some cases it's much easier overall to make a prosthesis after taking a cast impression of the surface where it will fit. The range of applications is startling, and covers literally the entire human body. We'll cover a few to illustrate the techniques.

Casting Materials

The first step is to make a cast of the part of the body where you want to apply a built-up feature. This produces a negative cast, into which you pour other material to make the positive cast on which you work for modification. One example is the ear, to obtain a base that you can build up into jug ears. Many industrial casting materials are caustic or toxic, and take too long to dry, which makes then unsuitable for human application.

Dental products are the safest to use, because they're designed to be non-irritating to the delicate mucous membranes of the mouth. They are also quicker setting than most other casting products. Local dental supply companies carry these, and are listed in the yellow pages.

There are three types of materials useful for casting: dental stone (a form of plaster), alginates, and synthetic rubbers, and all are available from dental supply houses. Dental stone is cheapest, alginates more expensive, and rubber compounds the most expensive. Rubber compounds provide the best accuracy because they conform to surface contours best, dental stone is least accurate, and alginates are in between.

Dental stone is a fine-grained, very quick-setting casting plaster. Its one drawback is that the process involves an "exothermic reaction," producing heat as it sets. Dental stone products become hot when setting, and require a couple of simple precautions to avoid discomfort or injury.

Make up only small amounts, an ounce or less. This keeps the volume down in proportion to surface area, and dissipates heat faster than would be possible with larger quantities. Also apply the material in thin layers, building it up gradually to the thickness you need. A thin layer generates less heat, and dissipates it faster. Setting time varies with the temperature of the water: the colder the water, the longer the working time. Typical working time is three to ten minutes. Overall, dental stone is best for the positive cast.

A faster setting type of material is alginate, and the type obtainable from a dental supply house sets in about three minutes. There are actually several alginate materials available, and setting times vary up to about six minutes. Mixing alginates with ice water extends setting time, as cold slows the chemical reaction.[1]

The drawback with alginate is that it's for one-time use, as pouring several applications of plaster will destroy it. Alginate is also only good for casting while wet. Once dry, it loses all flexibility, and you have to chip it off to get your cast free.

There are two types of synthetic rubbers: polysulfides and silicon rubber. Setting time for both is about 7-8 minutes. Both have two parts: rubber and catalyst, and you mix them according to instructions just before use. The major advantages of these types are flexibility, accuracy in reproducing skin pores, and the ability to make several positive casts from each.

These rubbers come in several degrees of hardness, and for our applications the softest are best because you need flexibility. The human ear, for example, has many compound curves, and removing the positive casting from the mold can be very difficult if the material is hard to work. This is why soft and stretchy material is best.

Casting Techniques

Making a cast of a body part is more craftsmanship than anything else. You have to use care in mixing the materials and applying them, and this section will walk you through the techniques.

When making a cast of a part of the body or face, an important first step is to apply a thin and even coat of Vaseline as a release agent. This will prevent sticking to the skin or to hairs, and make removal much easier. Keeping the release coat thin avoids masking fine details, such as skin pores. If making a cast of the nose or ear, a wad of cotton in the orifices will keep the material from trickling into them.

Mix the material carefully, stirring it thoroughly to blend the catalyst and work out bubbles. Apply the material, preferably polysulfide or silicon rubber, with a brush or spatula, and allow it to set. Peel off the mold, then make your positive cast.

The positive cast should be dental stone, because silicon rubber tends to stick to itself unless you apply a coat of release agent. This isn't necessary if you use dental stone, and the plaster will result in a hard positive cast that will retain its shape when you begin to alter its contours.

Once you have your positive cast, which should be a reproduction of the feature you want to alter, you build it up with clay. Not just any clay will do. You need a high-grade molding clay, known as "plastalene" or "plasticine," available in art supply stores. These are oil-base clays, which do not dry out and which release easily from the final mold you'll make once the contours of the remodeled feature are satisfactory.[2]

Apply the clay and build it up to the shape you want. You may need some sculptor's tools, such as spatulas of varying sizes and shapes. Smooth out the contours to make release easier, because nicks and dents will impede separation.

Another way is to use wax for both the positive casting and for the contouring material. Wax has the advantage of being reusable, and you can repair dents and other irregularities with a heated sculpting tool. Wax also releases very well from the mold, although soft waxes are somewhat fragile. Hard wax is more difficult to work, but the advantage is that it's more rugged and longer-lasting.

When you're satisfied with the new contours of your positive mold, you're ready for the final step, which will vary with the feature you're altering.

Jug Ears

The first step is to make a negative cast of the original ear. Use thin plastic sheeting to protect the hair around the ear, cutting out a center section to fit around the ear. You then apply silicon rubber to the ear, first plugging the ear canal with cotton or clay to prevent the rubber from dripping into it.

Once the silicon rubber casting has set, remove it carefully from the ear. Pour dental stone into the mold cavity and let it dry to produce a positive casting. Strip off the silicon rubber mold carefully, without tearing it, as you may want to use it again.

The final step is to paint layers of latex onto the positive of the ear in thin layers, allowing each layer to dry thoroughly before painting on the next. Build up the latex layers until you have an ear that looks like the one you want. Peel it off carefully, as latex tears easily. Dust the latex with a thin coat of translucent powder or talc to mask the sticky surface. When applying to the subject's ears, be especially careful to avoid folding the edges under.

Matching the latex to the subject's skin tone is the final step. The quick and dirty way is to put the ear on the subject with spirit gum, then use make-up cremes to match the skin tone. The problem with this is that it's likely to be a one-time method, because many make-up cremes have Vaseline or another petroleum base, and these attack the latex. If you decide to use make-up, apply the right shade, blending it in with surrounding skin, and finish with a layer of translucent powder.

Another way is to paint the ear, using a latex or acrylic base paint. The problem with this method is that paint doesn't necessarily match skin texture, and may peel.

The best way is to mix dye into the latex to produce a prosthesis that requires no additional color to blend with the subject's skin. You may have to make several tries until you get the color right, because the color darkens as latex cures.[3] You'll still have to do a final touch-up to blend the latex edges smoothly into the skin.

Teeth

For stage and film use, this technique allows producing vampire teeth and other outlandish effects, but for normal appearance changing, it's enough to enlarge the teeth slightly or to fill in gaps between them. You can also reduce the prominence of large frontal incisors by making the other teeth larger to match.

Making teeth prostheses is very complex, and requires a negative and positive mold, as well as a lot of hand-finishing. The first step is to make a cast of the teeth and gums, using a dental impression plate to support the casting material.[4]

Synthetic rubber compound is best, although the most expensive, because it's easy to use. Mix, pour into impression tray, insert into your mouth and bite down. Allow time for it to set, then remove. Use dental stone to make a positive cast of your teeth and gums, using a spatula and applying a small amount into each tooth cavity to make sure each fills in with plaster. Pour more plaster on top of the impression mold. Pour another quantity of plaster into a rough mold made of wax paper to produce a plaster disc about an inch high by 2½" wide. This will be the base. Now invert your impression mold, plaster and all, onto the plaster disc before the plaster sets. Allow to dry. This will produce the positive of the teeth, which you then reshape by adding clay to build up the desired areas. Make sure the clay goes right to the gum line.

Now you need an impression of the reshaped teeth. Coat the clay with a thin film of petroleum jelly, then make another cast with the impression plate. Once the synthetic rubber cures, remove the positive casting and peel the clay from it.

The next step is to make the prosthesis, using both the new impression and the positive casting to form the inside of the new teeth. The material you'll use is acrylic casting material called "temporary bridge resin," available from dental supply outlets. Use a shade to match the real teeth.

This is quick-setting resin, so you'll have to work fast. Squeeze some acrylic powder into each tooth cavity in the impression, then add resin and mix thoroughly, making sure there's enough mixture to run up to the gum line. Press the plaster positive into the impression, hard enough to cause the acrylic to flow, but not so hard as to push the teeth into the bottom of the impression. This is the difficult part, because you have to do it by feel as well as by eye. Once it's in place, give it plenty of time to set. The prosthesis will be thin, and you don't want to risk tearing, breaking, or distorting it by applying any force before it's thoroughly cured.

Separate the positive and negative molds, and you'll have a set of caps for your teeth. Try them for fit. You'll find that there are sharp edges you'll have to remove with a set of hand files or a motorized Dremel Tool. Cut a notch in the center, between the two front teeth, for the frenum, the thin strip of tissue that connects the inside of your lip to your gum.

Try for fit again. File or sand any rough or high spots, so that the prosthesis fits comfortably. Once you attain a perfect fit, you're ready for the final step. Use acrylic paints or epoxy with added coloring to fill in any gaps and bubbles, and to paint the gums to the right shade to match your gums.

Noses

The technique for producing a nose prosthesis is similar to the one for teeth, but you don't need a dental impression plate. Put cotton or wax into each nostril to prevent the silicon rubber from flowing into them, and use a spatula to coat the nose with the material. To prevent drip, use several coats, unless you want to dip your nose into a small paper cup of material.

Make your positive cast, build up the exterior to produce a bulbous nose or whatever other modification you want, and make another negative cast of the newly contoured proboscis. Use the negative and positive casts to make the prosthesis, using foam latex as the material. Foam latex is available from make-up and other suppliers, and is a variant of liquid latex, with a filler added.

In this case, you may wish to mix flesh coloring with the latex before casting. Matching paint of any sort to skin is more difficult and the paint can crack and peel because your nose prosthesis will be flexible. Finish the new nose by trimming to fit, and use spirit gum to apply it.

Latex Foreskins

This unusual type of prosthesis has been in use for some time, although largely undocumented. Some applications are for circumcised males who want to be able to pass for normal when visiting a foreign country, and members of religious minorities who want to pass a drop-your-pants inspection in places such as Yugoslavia, where the recent strife between Christian Serbs and Muslim Bosnians has led to ethnic repression. A recent application was to allow actors in an X-rated film to appear genuine down to the last detail, because the film's setting was in ancient Greece and to appear authentic, the actors had to appear intact.[5]

The basic technique of producing a fake foreskin is to make a thick condom-like prosthesis to slip over the penis and cover the denuded glans. The first step is to make a silicon rubber cast of an intact penis, and use this mold to cast a plaster positive. The intact penis used for a pattern should be close in size and proportions to the trimmed one you wish to re-cover. The closer the fit, the easier it will be to put on and remove the prosthesis, and the more natural it will appear.

If you plan to wear the fake foreskin for more than a few hours, you'll probably want to provide for urination. Insert a straw into the urethra before making the first casting, to allow for a hole in the foreskin's tip. If you forget this step, cut a slit in the end of the finished foreskin prosthesis with a razor knife.

There are two ways of fabricating the foreskin prosthesis. One requires coating the plaster penis with vegetable jelly, such as K-Y, as a release agent, and painting it with liquid latex with flesh tone blended in. Use many thin coats to retain as much skin detail as possible, and make it long enough to reach the hair line. Try to make the rearmost section thinner, to avoid a hard line of demarcation between the latex and the shaft skin. The result should be at least five times as thick as a condom to simulate the thickness of a genuine foreskin. When it's finished, allow to cure thoroughly and peel it from the positive pattern. This device will have a perfect reproduction of skin texture on the inside, but the outside will tend to lose the pores and fine wrinkles.

The second method is better because of superior reproduction of skin texture, and requires pouring a coat of flesh-colored latex into the silicone rubber penis mold, making sure it spreads evenly. When it's dry, pour another coat into the mold, to build up the thickness of the latex foreskin. Try to make the rearmost section thinner, to avoid a hard line of demarcation between the latex and the shaft skin. Allow to cure thoroughly and peel it from the inside of the mold.

To use the foreskin prosthesis, lubricate the inside with K-Y or other vegetable jelly to allow it to slip on, and use spirit gum to anchor the rear edge. Urination may be a problem, because the latex may not stretch enough to clear the meatus, and it may well be necessary to sit down for this function, wiping the tip carefully afterward.

A commercially available artificial foreskin, the "Sensitizer," is available from Travel Mate, PO Box 66414, Houston, TX 77006. Cost is $10 for a package of four.

Casting Fills A Need

Although casting prostheses is more elaborate than other kinds of make-up, it's a time-saver. Having a prosthesis ready-made allows applying it quickly, unlike conventional make-up techniques which require careful building up with wax or putty. A casting is also re-usable, important if you need more than one use.

Notes

1. *The Technique of the Professional Make-up Artist*, Vincent J. R. Kehoe, Boston, Focal Press, 1985, p. 167.
2. *Ibid.*, p. 172.
3. *Ibid.*, p. 188.
4. *Three-Dimensional Make-up*, Lee Baygan, NY, Watson-Guptill Publications, 1982, pp. 138-140.
5. *Uncut* Magazine, January, 1993, pp. 20-24.

Chapter Ten

A POCKET DISGUISE KIT

In some instances, you may need a small, light, and very portable disguise kit. (See Figure 10-1.) This can be as small as a plastic bag for pocket carry, or as comprehensive as a larger kit that fits only in an attaché case or tackle box. The size of the kit, and the selection of items, depend on individual requirements. A female won't need shaving gear, for example. Let's look at items we might consider including, and study their usefulness.

The Container can be almost anything. A plastic box or paper bag, practical although not elegant, is cheap but does the job. A plastic tackle box or a briefcase are more durable and convenient, but more costly and bulky. When choosing a container, the only serious requirements are that it mustn't be cumbersome, and must fit into the situation. An attaché case, for example, would be out of place if you're wearing a repairman's overalls. Likewise, a toolbox wouldn't fit with a three-piece suit. A simple container that fits easily inside another is an excellent choice. A flat box that can go inside a grocery bag, tool box, or attaché case serves the purpose very well.

Comb, hairbrush, and fake hair disguise the hair. A quick change in hair style can work wonders. So does a wig, false mustache, or sideburns.

Hair spray is optional, but it helps hold a radically different hair style in place. However, it's awkward to carry a large can of hair spray in your kit, so you may be better off spraying your hair at home. A wet comb will soften the hair spray, allowing you to re-style your hair when you need it.

Scissors are useful for a quick and severe hair trim, or as a preliminary to shaving a real beard, mustache, or pair of sideburns.

Disposable safety razors belong in every disguise kit, along with a small tube of shaving cream. These are lighter and cheaper than an electric shaver, and the battery won't go dead at a critical moment.

A roll-up hat is a must. Donning a hat of any sort changes the silhouette radically, and is so easy and quick, that a hat is a vital component of any disguise kit. The most important point about a hat is that you can put it on or take it off in public without attracting the attention you would by cutting your hair or applying a wig or false mustache.

Adhesive for false sideburns or a mustache. Spirit gum is the mainstay of theatrical people, but any adhesive that doesn't irritate your skin, even double-face tape, will do. For those lucky people with skin like armor plate, contact cement will work in a pinch.

A mirror helps you to don a disguise. Don't depend on mirrors always being available in public places. You'd attract attention putting on a false mustache in a public toilet, or looking at your reflection in a shop window. A small mirror with a folding base, possibly with a battery-powered light, should suit every situation.

Foundation to match your skin is important if you plan to use other make-up or putty to create bumps and spots on your face. Putty, although flesh-colored, probably won't match your skin tone exactly, no matter how much you blend it in with your fingers.

Liner stick is for creating age lines. This is quick and easy to apply, but absolutely requires a mirror.

Black wax crayon is for creating the illusion of a missing tooth.

Paper towels. Applying and removing skin creams is messy, and you'll need to wipe your fingers.

Wash-N-Dry moist towelettes, available in most pharmacies and supermarkets, clean stubborn stains from your face and hands.

Eyeglasses, either regular or sunglasses, are instant disguises. Like hats, putting them on attracts no notice. You may want several styles, and even a pair of mirror sunglasses in your kit.

This short list cannot cover all situations, and you'll want to add other items as the need arises. The main point about a pocket disguise kit is that the contents must be quick and easy to apply.

Select each item with care, to obtain shades that match your skin tone as closely as possible. Don't order items and throw them into your kit without first trying them. Creating an effective disguise requires both selection and practice, and you'll have to experiment to find what's best for you.

Ordering a make-up kit and experimenting with each item, to weed out those less useful to you, is the best way to go about it. Weeding out is essential, because simply carrying a wide assortment of cremes and foundations to cover every possible use makes for a large, heavy, and cumbersome kit.

Sources are varied. A list of sources for various disguise items is included in Appendix IV. You may also want to buy over-the-counter from a local supplier, which you can find in the yellow pages.

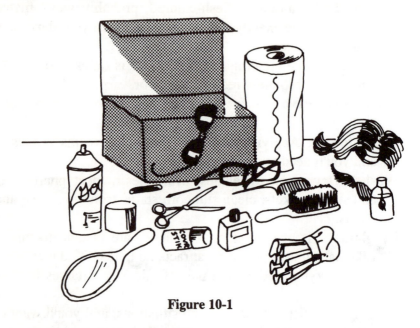

Figure 10-1

A pocket disguise kit should fit into a concealable container. A complete kit, like this one, has more than you'll normally need.

Chapter Eleven

DISGUISING THE VOICE

Disguising the voice can take several dimensions. First, there's the basic pitch, which the person can change with conscious effort, speaking in a deeper than normal tone. Next are harmonics caused by resonances in the throat and mouth. There are several ways of changing these, and all involve inserting something into the mouth or nose. Nose plugs constricting the nostrils will change resonance, giving the voice a higher sound. Stuffing cotton into the cheeks changes both voice and facial contours. Speech patterns and accents are characteristics that require constant conscious effort to change. Finally, there are electronic devices that change the voice's pitch.

Speech Prosthetics

Tongue position affects the voice, and keeping a marble or other small object under the tongue also changes the harmonics. There are also false palates for this purpose. These plastic or rubber devices aren't commonly available.

With slight mechanical ability, it's possible to produce your own. For this, you need a cast of your palate, made with modeling clay. Yes, it tastes awful, but it's non-toxic. The next step is to make a mold of the cast, using ordinary plaster. The final step is to make the false palate itself, using silicon rubber.

Silicon rubber is made by both General Electric and Dow Chemical, and is available locally from plastic supply houses. The type for casting is the two-part mixture that consists of the rubber and a catalytic agent. It's important to let the rubber casting cure completely before inserting it into the mouth, as some curing agents are toxic.

Caulking and sealing agents labeled "silicon rubber" are available in hardware stores aren't suitable for this purpose because they do not contain a "release agent" and they stick to the mold. These are single-part materials packed in tubes, and are easily identifiable by a strong acetic acid odor.

Making the false palate properly is mostly trial-and-error. Each false palate requires hand-fitting, and its thickness will determine the change in harmonics. You may have to make several palates before you get the effect you want.

When you complete your first casting, insert it and speak into a tape recorder. Compare the result with a tape of your normal voice. If the effect isn't enough, try a thicker insert.

Electronic Voice Modifiers

There are several small and portable electronic devices that change the voice's pitch. These are available locally in various "spy shops" and by mail-order. Advertisements for various electronic devices are in the classified sections of magazines such as *Mechanix Illustrated*.

Voice-changers cost between $90 and $300 retail. Their effectiveness depends on the listener, and how familiar he is with your voice. A voice pitch changer won't remove an accent, or change speech patterns, and if your manner of speaking is distinctive, you'll find that just changing the pitch of your voice won't go far in disguising it.[1]

Voice Training and Development

You can also study books on developing the voice.[2] Some are of limited value, dealing only with projecting the voice, a technique useful for acting, public speaking, and commanding troops. These techniques are less important today than they were a century ago, when public-address systems didn't exist.

Accents

A more effective method of disguising the voice is to assume an accent, whether an ethnic one, or one from a foreign language. Another type is the regional accent. With enough effort, you can assume the accent you choose. It's not as easy as it may seem at first, though. Accents can be complex, involving slurring consonants and breaking up the syntax. Adding vowels to the ends of words does not make an Italian accent, despite a superficial impression.

Regional American accents are not too difficult for an American to assume. Foreign accents are another matter. A British accent is relatively easy, although many Americans do not realize that Britain also has regional accents. A London accent sounds quite different from a North Country or West Country accent, and it's difficult for a foreigner to distinguish between them. There are also class differences in British speech, with the upper socio-economic groups speaking very differently from the way working class people do. These distinctions can be important. Passing yourself off as an Englishmen to an American who has never been to the British Isles is relatively easy, but trying to fool a British subject is much harder. Claiming to have been born and raised in London, while speaking with a Manchester accent, is like an American with a Southern drawl presenting himself as a New Yorker.

You may remember a short-lived TV cop show, *Eischeid*, starring Joe Don Baker as the New York City Police Department's Chief of Detectives. Baker, with his thick Southern accent, did not fit the part of a New Yorker with a Jewish-sounding name. Baker's soft-sounding speech did not sound like a New York accent, with its crisp vowels and clicking consonants. The discrepancies go further than vowels and consonants. No New Yorker would use the Southern regional phrase, "Ya done good," that characterized Baker's Eischeid.

Some foreign accents are very difficult for an American to simulate. For example, the soft French "J"s and gutteral "R"s are serious obstacles, as is the sharp "U." American speakers are also unaccustomed to the fruity dipthongs of Czech, Russian, and other Slavic tongues. An American won't be able to duplicate them without extensive practice.

Unfortunately, learning a foreign language in school isn't much help. Most Americans who learn a European language can't ever pass themselves off as natives if they visit that country. Asian languages are even more difficult to imitate, but there's no purpose in trying, because if you're Caucasian you would never pass for an Asian, no matter how well you speak the language and mimic the accent.

A few private schools, such as Berlitz, do a very good job of teaching foreign languages, and this might be worthwhile for someone willing to spend the time and money required. A better and cheaper way is to enroll in a speech class at a local community college. Typically, a speech course teaches students the movements of the mouth necessary to produce various sounds, and how to put them together to produce correct speech.

Speech classes are often remedial, aimed at those who have foreign or regional accents, but the techniques are useful for imitating an accent as well as suppressing one. In fact, they are the same, because speech classes actually teach students the accent of the area where they are taught.

Speech Patterns

Altering the manner of speech also disguises the voice. We all know that there's a difference in speech patterns between people who have various levels of education. It's easier, though, for an educated person to break up his syntax and introduce grammatical errors and mispronunciations than the other way around. Again, the key is practice.

Another way to change your voice is to alter your hearing. Plugging your ears makes your voice sound differently to you, as well as changing the character of external sounds. The natural tendency is to compensate for the difference by changing your speech. You may speak more loudly than when unplugged, or stress high-pitched sounds such as "S"s and "Z"s.

The best way to plug your ears inconspicuously is to use the soft, flesh-colored ear plugs available in pharmacies and department stores. These are made of soft wax or plastic which you can shape to fit. Cotton also works, although its white color makes it conspicuous. At all costs, don't place extremely small objects into your ears, because you may not be able to remove them.

Although altering your hearing won't make a substantial difference in your voice, when you combine this with a conscious effort to change your speech pattern, you'll add to the effect of your disguise. Learning and practicing take time.

Tape Recorders for Practice

The first step is to obtain a tape recording of someone of the same sex speaking in the accent you want to simulate. The next is practice, practice, practice! Using a tape recorder is essential, because the way you hear your voice is not the way it sounds to others. Try various accents, as you'll find some easier to assume than others. With many hours of practice, you'll perfect your adopted accent.

One problem with adopted accents and speech patterns is that, under emotional stress, you may find yourself reverting to your native accent. This can be jarring to the listener, and will probably give you away.

Speech Defects

What we call "speech defects" overlap with accents and speech patterns. Some people consider poor grammar and an uneducated manner of speaking a speech defect, while others limit the definition to stuttering and structural defects in the speech organs. Correcting structural defects, such as a cleft palate and other deformities, requires surgery and is definitely not a do-it-yourself project. However, stuttering, which affects between 2% and 5% of the population, depending on which study you choose to believe, is possible to modify without medical attention.

Nobody really knows why some people stutter and others don't. Psychiatrists and psychologists have offered various theories, mostly linked to early childhood experiences. Whatever the causes may be, it's clear that eliminating stuttering increases the effectiveness of a disguise because it eliminates one obvious identifier.

There is a self-treatment method for stuttering.[3] This falls into the category of "behavior therapy," and while it doesn't always work, it costs almost nothing to use and takes very little time. The basic method consists of relaxation exercises, and practicing breathing and speaking in short phrases.

Lisping is another speech problem that you can suppress. The basic technique is similar to the methods you use to correct stuttering. Practice consists of reading aloud words containing the letter "S" while thrusting the jaw forward and pronouncing the "S"s clearly. As with stuttering, the cost and time needed are so little that it's worthwhile for anyone with a lisp to try the behavioral method first, before spending time and money on a doctor or psychiatrist.[4]

There are other ways to disguise the voice, simulating certain characteristics. One fairly common characteristic is hoarseness, from a cold or cough, or from excessive drinking — what's come to be known as "whiskey voice." Acquiring hoarseness is only a matter of shouting, preferably in an isolated place, until the strain causes your voice to become hoarse. You'll end up with a sore throat, but the result may be worth the discomfort.

A quicker and less rigorous way is simply to speak in a loud whisper. Many people will assume that your throat is irritated, and you can help the illusion by pointing to your throat when someone asks you to repeat what you said or shows difficulty in hearing you.

The voice is only one dimension of human behavior, and learning to modify it can help a lot to increase the effectiveness of a disguise.

Notes

1. Voice changers are available from several sources:

Eavesdropping Detection Equipment
PO Box 337
Buffalo, NY 14226
Phone: (716) 691-3476
Fax: (716) 691-0604

EDE provides a digital, battery-powered voice changer that goes over the phone's mouthpiece, and includes a button-activated barking dog simulator.

Operative Supply
PO Box 2343
Atlantic Beach, NC 28512
Phone: (919) 726-1582
Operative Supply provides three models of electronic voice changers. One is a small digital voice changer powered by one 9-volt battery. Another, powered by four AA batteries, installs between the handset and phone on two-piece telephones, and provides 16 voice changing levels. The third is a telephone with built-in voice changer.

Productive Electronic Products
PO Box 930024
Norcross, GA 30093
Phone: (404) 938-0381
PEP makes the "vocomask," a battery-powered device that goes between the handset and body of a two-piece telephone, and digitally changes the voice's pitch.

2. Richard Sharretts, *Command Voice*, Harrisburg, PA, Stackpole Company, 1973, and Dr. Morton Cooper, *Change Your Voice: Change Your Life*, NY, Barnes & Noble Books, 1984.
3. Nathan H. Azrin, Ph. D., and R. Gregory Nunn, Ph. D., *Habit Control in a Day*, NY, Pocket Books, pp. 121-134.
4. *Ibid.*, pp. 144-146.

Chapter Twelve

MANNERISMS, HABITS, AND GAIT

As pointed out in the make-up chapter, changing appearance alone does not make a complete disguise. If you're trying to play a role, cosmetic change is only the first step. Clothing must fit the role, as well as speech patterns and other behavior. If you're trying to avoid being recognized by people who know you, your gait and mannerisms may give you away even if you don't speak. There are techniques for modifying behavior patterns to impede recognition or to play a role. Some are simple; others are more involved.

Walk

Changing a limp to a normal walk may be very difficult, depending on the degree of impairment. Shoe inserts may help, but this is a problem that often doesn't yield to simple measures. Time-consuming physical rehabilitative therapy may be necessary, and sometimes this isn't enough.

On the other hand, simulating a limp can be as simple as keeping a pebble in one shoe. A less uncomfortable way is to buy a set of shoe inserts, or lifts, and use only one. This will produce a definite limp, but if you have to run, an insert can be a severe handicap.

Some people have characteristic walks. Some tend to crouch while walking, with arms held out from the sides. Others have a rolling walk, as if they were on the deck of a ship. Ex-convicts are sometimes conspicuous by the struts they acquired in prison. It's possible to modify these habits by intensive practice, but for temporary purposes the quick way is to use a prop, both to change the stance and as a reminder to walk differently.

The person who walks in a crouch can suppress the habit by holding the arms out and carrying something heavy, such as a toolbox, in one hand. The weight will drag the arm down, and to retain body symmetry the other arm will come down as well. The weight is a reminder to walk upright, because carrying a heavy object is easier with the back straight.

A rolling walk is harder to suppress. A ruler or dowel taped to the skin along the spine serves as a reminder, but this isn't always practical while wearing disguise. The situation may require sitting or bending, making the ruler under clothing impractical. It's best to practice extensively with the ruler taped in place, but to remove it when actually playing the role.

Speech

Certain speech habits properly belong in the category we call "mannerisms." Some people characteristically begin every sentence with "Well..." or punctuate their words with "y'know" several times in each sentence. Others characteristically use profanity. It's easy for people to remain unaware of their distinctive speech patterns, especially if many of their associates express themselves the same way.

The list of speech mannerisms is quite long, and many people have them, even well-educated people. Some mannerisms are quite subtle, and are grammatically correct, but are still atypical and characteristic expressions that identify the speaker sight unseen, such as on the telephone. Some of these speech mannerisms and pet phrases are: "the bottom line," "okay," "sure," "no way," "it doesn't compute," and "in other words." People who are addicted to using such phrases repeatedly in their speech will retain a clearly identifiable speech pattern.

Speech mannerisms also help identify regional and cultural origins. "No way" is characteristic of the Western states, hardly heard East of the Mississippi. "Y'all" is Southern speech, while "heyyy, heyyy," is stereotypical low-class New Yorkese. Some New Yorkers, especially those from the Bronx, begin their sentences with "Uhhhh..."

Speech patterns can cause severe problems for some people who aren't necessarily trying to avoid recognition by people they know. Someone who settles in a Western state and claims that he's from Florida, yet has a heavy New England accent or speech pattern, will alert anyone familiar with the way Floridians speak that he's not genuine. On the other hand, a fellow New Yorker or Bostonian may recognize the speech pattern immediately, despite a conscious effort to develop a Southern drawl.

Eliminating these mannerisms takes conscious effort over a long time, and many practice sessions with a tape recorder. One way to begin is to describe, each evening, the events of the day, then play the tape while listening carefully. Speech patterns will become evident. The speaker can work to change them, making another recording after auditing the first one.

Another way, more expensive and time-consuming, is to join a local chapter of the Toastmasters Club. The new member will quickly discover that he's not the only one with speech mannerisms, and that others are even worse. He'll be surprised to find out how many people, instead of saying a sentence in one bite, utter fragments punctuated by several "uhs" and "ahs." It often takes months or years, but many people have been able to modify and improve their speech patterns after joining Toastmasters.

Habits

Many people have characteristic habits, such as nail biting, hair stroking or pulling, or scratching themselves. Nobody has been able to prove what causes such habit patterns to develop, but they've given psychologists and psychiatrists many happily profitable hours "treating" people who have come to them seeking a "cure." Possibly the greatest sufferers are those with tics, also known as "habit spasms." These are muscle movements, some involving large muscles of the body, but more often facial muscles. These "nervous twitches" are a social handicap as well as a means of recognition, and they cause distress to those who have them.

Suppressing these highly visible means of identification can be very difficult indeed. Unfortunately, many have gone to psychiatrists, and have found themselves undergoing rigorous treatments, including electroshock therapy in some instances, in an effort to get "cured."[1]

There's a strong tendency among psychiatrists and other doctors to try one treatment after another, all at the patient's expense, of course, until they find one that seems to work. Although this may stem from genuine eagerness to help the patient, it's still the patient who pays the bills and takes the treatments, including suffering serious side effects.

The less formidable methods of dealing with these habits —
psychotherapy and psychoanalysis — generally don't work well
either. Although without the serious side effects of electroshock, they can and often do produce serious anxiety. They're
also often so drawn-out that they begin to appear like an illness
in themselves. Add to this the fact that there are many different
"schools" of psychotherapy and psychoanalysis, and we have a
disastrous situation. A patient who finds that one doctor is not
helping him will often go to another who uses different methods. The second one is no more likely than the first to get results, and the patient will try another and another, as long as his
money lasts.

Some drugs have been successful in treating habits and
mannerisms. Tranquilizers often have a calming effect, while
others work in ways that are yet unknown. Haloperidol works to
suppress spasms of the large muscles, but not the smaller ones.
Clonidine is sometimes effective against "Tourette's Syn-
drome," a severe habit spasm disorder that sometimes produces
bizarre tics and vocalizations. Again, nobody really knows how
or why. Drugs are cheaper than long-term psychotherapy, and
often it's possible to judge whether a drug is helpful before suffering permanent side effects.

All of these drugs have side effects, which can be serious,
depending on the dosage and the individual. Haloperidol, for
example, can cause blurring of vision, drowsiness, and lethargy,
all of which are serious handicaps for the person who drives a
car. Stopping the drug will cause these side effects to vanish.
However, extended use can produce "tardive dyskinesia," a
condition which ironically resembles tics with its uncontrol-
lable muscle spasms. Unfortunately, this is a physical nervous
disorder that is irreversible once it occurs. Stopping the drug
will not stop the symptoms.[2]

There are ways of suppressing habits, at least temporarily.
The basic tactic is to consciously substitute another movement

for the one suppressed. For example, facial tics will yield to gum chewing, sometimes for hours. The person with facial tics finds that the rhythmic movement of the jaw while chewing will eliminate the tics that are otherwise so noticeable.

The principle of substitution is the core of the method of habit suppression and control explained in the book, *Habit Control in a Day*.[3] With conscious effort and practice, it's possible to contract a muscle that pulls in the opposite direction, thus suppressing the visible symptom.

Suppressing habits and mannerisms crosses over into the area of body image modification, in which there are definite psychological benefits that go with the physical changes. The person ends up feeling better about himself, and gains in self-confidence. The method used is essentially a disguise, but the purpose is not as much to deceive as to improve body image. It's an internal change as well as an external one. It's also a real change, not a merely cosmetic one.

Notes

1. Lother B. Kalinowsky, M. D., and Paul D. Hoch, M. D., *Shock Treatment, Psychosurgery, and Other Somatic Treatments in Psychiatry*, NY, Grune & Stratton, 1952, p. 203.
2. James W. Long, M. D., *The Essential Guide to Prescription Drugs*, NY, Harper & Row, 1980, pp. 344-345.
3. Nathan H. Azrin, Ph. D., and R. Gregory Nunn, Ph. D., *Habit Control in a Day*, NY, Pocket Books. This book is essentially a do-it-yourself guide to modifying bad habits. The title implies that it can all happen in one day, but realistically it takes longer. The authors explain a program of habit control that the reader can begin at once, with positive results, but carrying it through takes more than a single day, and a more realistic time frame is several weeks. The book

is worth reading, because its methods work, but it's unfortunate that such a book must be flawed by a title that is
mostly hype.

Chapter Thirteen

BLENDING WITH THE CROWD

An important aspect of disguise is blending into a crowd or locale, which does not necessarily require make-up, false beards, or any radical change in appearance. Blending takes in two basic principles:

1. Fitting in with the crowd or locale.
2. Not doing anything to stand out from the crowd.

These principles are complementary, and when you work to satisfy one, you're well on your way to fulfilling the other. Let's look at specific examples:

A detective conducting a surveillance will want to remain unnoticed by his subject. This doesn't mean an appearance change, because the odds are overwhelming that the subject does not know the detective, and would not recognize him if they came face to face. The detective merely wants to assure that the subject does not begin to notice him.

A criminal fleeing the scene of a major felony does not want to spoil his getaway with an accident, or attract attention by excessive speed or weaving in and out. Typical suspect behavior, once clear of the immediate area, is to drive at the same speed as other traffic, and to blend in with it.[1]

Chameleon Disguise

What Edmond MacInaugh calls "chameleon disguise" is fitting into a situation, not impersonating a specific person.[2] It means dressing and acting like one of a class of people, not a specific person. Mail carriers, police officers, window-washers, porters, repairmen, construction workers, and vagrants are people most of us pass by without a second glance. In some areas, military uniforms are common, because of nearby military bases.

Some police officers have had extensive experience in assuming generic disguises. Shadowing and surveillance demand fading into the background, and this requires attention to detail as well as basic acting skill. One detail some inexperienced officers overlook is that even dirty clothing, such as those worn by a vagrant, isn't enough if the officer wears shiny black shoes.

Posing as a vagrant or wino takes more than ragged clothing, depending on the closeness of the inspection you must pass. A decoy, waiting to be "rolled" by a mugger must look the part but he doesn't have to pass inspection by many people. Several days' beard and a noticeable body odor help perfect the disguise.

Motor Vehicles

Many police detectives and plainclothesmen for years thought that they could avoid attracting attention and alerting the suspects by driving unmarked vehicles when on stake-out or surveillance. An "unmarked" vehicle is simply the same model vehicle as a patrol car, but in plain colors and without a light bar on top. They remained unaware that street-wise suspects soon learned to recognize detective cars because they were typically low-end four-door cars, with minimal chrome and trim, and plain blackwall tires. Such a vehicle, especially with two bulky men with short haircuts in the front seat, almost screams "cops."

Today, savvy plainclothes officers take advantage of this stereotype. While detectives assigned to homicide units drive plain "company cars" to their assignments, detectives on surveillances and stake-outs choose anything but. They may drive confiscated vehicles, perhaps a Corvette, or if they want to appear less racy, a cheap Toyota. Few American agencies use foreign cars for patrol vehicles, and foreign makes connote anything but "cop."

There are two components to vehicular disguise: blending and avoiding. Blending means choosing a vehicle of a common make, model, and color for the area. For example, a high-priced make would fit into a wealthy area, and a trashy, old, low-end car with dents and rust blends into the milieu in a run-down area. Pick-up trucks or vans are popular in some areas, while standard sedans fit into other locales.

Color can be important. In northern climates, almost any color is as good as another, unless the color choice is chartreuse with pink stripes. In torrid areas, the most popular color is white.

Props can be important. A baby seat in a car used in a family neighborhood fits right into the picture. In a tourist area, an out-of-state license plate sends the message that the car is a tourist vehicle. A camper or van also fits into the tourist role.

Avoiding anything that makes you stand out is the other aspect. A pair of foam dice hanging from the mirror is easy to see in the rear-view when you're shadowing someone. Bumper stickers are another no-no.[3] Driving through a Jewish neighborhood with a sticker that says "HITLER WAS RIGHT!" will bring all sorts of unwanted attention. Any sticker with an obscene slogan will be conspicuous. So will a sticker saying "I'M THE NRA." You may find that someone has broken into your vehicle looking for guns.

A heavy coat of dust or road grime helps the disguise, especially if the vehicle is cheap and a few years old. Dirt and road grime would be out of place on a luxury car, though.

Another point, especially important to fugitives but also to ordinary citizens, is not attracting the attention of the police. A "muscle car," such as a Corvette or Jaguar, always attracts attention from speed cops, and if you're slightly heavy-footed, you'll soon find flashing lights in your rear-view mirror. If you drive a Yugo, Toyota or Chevy Sprint, cops will give you only a passing glance unless your driving style is outlandish.

Small details are important, as well, because they can lead to police stops. It's literally true that you can drive across the country with a forged or expired driver's license, or even no license at all. But if a police officer stops you, whatever the reason, his first step will be to ask to see your driver's license and vehicle registration.

A police officer must have "probable cause" to stop you, and this isn't limited to a screeching, smoking-tires departure from the scene of a bank robbery. It also can mean a trivial infraction such as a burned-out headlight or brake light, or excessive exhaust smoke. A traffic stop for any reason gives the officer further opportunity to scrutinize you, and if you appear nervous, this will further arouse his suspicions. He'll also be looking for anything that seems out of place, and this can be an expensive attaché case on the seat of an old car.

Police aren't the only problem, especially for an honest citizen. Car thieves abound, and you might find your expensive car stereo stolen, or the car itself may disappear if it's a model that attracts thieves. The general rule is that car thieves steal late-model luxury or sports cars, for resale or spare parts. They rarely steal older vehicles, or cheaper models, because the cash return isn't worth their while. This is why it's usually best to drive a low-end, slightly shabby vehicle to avoid attention from both cops and robbers.

Premises

You may want to disguise where you live, or disguise temporary quarters, such as those used for stationary surveillance. The trick here is to choose a room or apartment in an area where people are not curious about their neighbors. A relatively new apartment house is a good choice, especially if there's a high turn-over rate. In such places, people simply don't get to know their neighbors. Minimizing your exposure also means not entering or leaving at times when many other residents do. Avoiding the morning or afternoon rush hours, when people leave for work or return, avoids meeting neighbors. Another point is not having many visitors.

In some areas, many visitors to one apartment suggests "drug dealer" to the apartment manager. Another problem with visitors can be inadvertently parking in someone else's slot, which can provoke a confrontation. Some people become angry enough at someone taking their parking slots to physically damage the vehicle. Yet another possibility is that a person visiting you may be conspicuous because of a striking or outlandish appearance.

An obvious point is ethnicity. A minority member stands out in some areas, while a Caucasian would arouse curiosity renting in a ghetto. Choose living quarters where most residents are the same ethnicity as you, or where no single group predominates. Also, dress for the area, as covered in the last chapter.

Yet another point is your vehicle, if you have one. Make it a habit to park your vehicle several blocks away if you can, so that no neighbor sees it and connects you with it. This can be crucial because a neighbor can remember that a certain person was connected with a certain vehicle. What they don't see, they can't tell.

Surveillance

Carrying out a protracted surveillance can require more elaborate methods to avoid jeopardizing security. This is especially true of surveilling illegal activities. Police know that drug dealers operating from a house or apartment, for example, employ "look-outs." These are often teen-agers or pre-teens, instructed to notify the dealer of anyone or any vehicle loitering in the area. This makes it impossible for a surveillant to stand on the street corner reading a newspaper, or to lounge on a nearby bench. In such a case, no disguise proves effective, and it's important to remain out of sight. Renting premises nearby isn't always possible on short notice. Parking several blocks away and watching the premises with binoculars is one way of coping. Another is to use a special surveillance vehicle.

This is a truck, van, or camper which one officer drives up to the surveillance area, parks, and leaves. Inside the vehicle is a surveillance team which remains with the vehicle. Team members do not show themselves at all, remaining well back from the heavily-curtained windows. Some specially-equipped surveillance vans have a small closed-circuit TV camera built into a ventilation hatch at the top, allowing panoramic surveillance without disclosing the presence of the occupants.

Occupants must be careful not to do anything that would alert look-outs that the vehicle is occupied. Sudden movements could cause the vehicle to rock, and brushing against a window curtain would give a visual cue that someone's inside. During the hours of darkness, lighting a cigarette or using a flashlight to write a report would betray them. Also taboo are food and coffee runs, because people leaving and entering a supposedly parked vehicle would be an obvious give-away. There must be enough food and drink on board, as well as a chemical toilet, to make the occupants self-sufficient for at least 24 hours. Fortunately, this is cheap and easy to arrange.

Blending Works

Blending into the milieu is often easy at first, but carrying it out successfully for a protracted period takes concentration and attention to detail. In some situations, camouflage of some sort helps, and we'll study this in the next chapter.

Notes

1. *Law and Order*, October, 1992, p. 157.
2. *Disguise Techniques,* Edmond A. MacInaugh, Boulder, CO, Paladin Press, 1984, p. 29.
3. *Ibid.*, p. 33.

Chapter Fourteen

CAMOUFLAGE

Camouflage is the ultimate form of disguise, to blend in not with the crowd, but with your surroundings. Unfortunately, there's been a tremendous amount of misinformation about camouflage, and many forms of camouflage don't work in certain environments. Let's take a close look at what camouflage really is, to gain an understanding of what camouflage is not.

Camouflage: How it Works

Camouflage is suppressing any characteristics that make you stand out from your surroundings. As people see you with their senses, you can be conspicuous because of brightness, color, shape, and noise. We've all seen military "cammo" suits, with woodland or desert shades in broken patterns, which help blend into a rustic setting.[1] In winter, white snow suits blend with snow and ice. However, clothing is just the beginning.

Suppressing bright colors is equally important. Camouflage kits include face creams to darken the skin to match the setting. Night camouflage requires burned cork or a black or gray face cream to make exposed skin blend in with darkness. Bright and shiny objects don't belong in the open for successful camouflage. Bright buttons, name tags, cameras, and weapons also must be concealed or colored to match. A serious error some military observers make is using binoculars, because the large objective lenses reflect light and can cause a glint, revealing their positions. If it's necessary to use binoculars, use them under the shade of a tree or wall or deep inside a room away from windows, not in direct sunlight.

Suppressing characteristic shape is also important. No matter how well your cammos blend in with the environment, you'll be very visible if you stand against the skyline. Even close to the ground, it's better to remain partly concealed behind a bush or rock, so that an observer doesn't see the characteristic human shape.

Noise also betrays your position. Tape all keys and other metal objects. Be careful where you step, to avoid dislodging a rock or breaking a twig. If you must use a radio, make sure it has an earphone, not a speaker, or an incoming message will announce your location to anyone who hears it.

Another strategy to pass unnoticed in a rural setting is to appear to belong there. This is sometimes better than trying to be totally invisible, because it allows you free movement in the area. A farmer's overalls or jeans fit in much better than a three-piece suit.

Urban Camouflage

We can easily see that some types of "camouflage" are totally inappropriate in some environments. Green and brown pattern cammos in an urban setting make you stand out like a clown suit at a funeral.

The key is to wear apparel that suggests that you're a normal part of the setting. A street cleaner's outfit puts you beneath notice, as does a window washer's. Fortunately, the clothing needed for urban camouflage is dirt-cheap, and commonly available.[2]

Timing is important in a built-up area. Street cleaners, window washers, and mail carriers rarely work at night, and using one of these outfits for camouflage limits you to weekday daylight hours. For off-hours a set of chinos and a tool kit suggest that you're a repairman on an urgent call.

Making it Work

Together, camouflage and blending techniques will help make you invisible in almost any setting. The keys are choosing appropriate garb and acting the part.

Notes

1. Military-type "cammos" are available from:

SHOMER-TEC
PO Box 2039
Bellingham, WA 98227
Phone: (206) 733-6214
Fax: (206) 676-5248

2. Two sources for uniforms and work clothes are:

Broadway Costumes, Inc.
954 West Washington Blvd.
Fourth Floor
Chicago, IL 60607
Phone: (800) 397-3316
(312) 829-6400
Fax: (312) 829-8621

WearGuard Work Clothes
Longwater Drive
Norwell, MA 02061
Phone: (800) 388-3300

Chapter Fifteen

PLASTIC SURGERY

Plastic surgery is a growth industry in the United States, and today over one million Americans have some sort of cosmetic operation each year.[1] About 30% of those having plastic surgery come from families with less than $25,000/year incomes. About 35% have family incomes in the $25,000 to $50,000 bracket.[2] Men as well as women have plastic surgery done, because it's becoming more fashionable. Plastic surgery is a lucrative business. At the time of writing (1992), there are almost 4,000 members of the American Society of Plastic and Reconstructive Surgeons (ASPRS).

In every field, there are legends and misconceptions. In the field of firearms, for example, there are still some who believe that the .30-30 was once the U.S. Army cartridge, and that a silencer will work on a revolver. Some believe that computers are infallible, or that all police officers are as clean-cut, dedicated, and incorruptible as the stars of the old TV show *Adam-12*.

Part of the reason that legends persist is that few people have the opportunity or inclination to check them against known facts. There are few fields in which this is more true than plastic surgery, and this is why legends abound.

Fact vs. Fiction

Fiction writers add to the misinformation. While many describe the actions of their heroes in exacting detail, they also describe unreal situations and unworkable schemes, the products of their imaginations and not taken from the real world. For example, in one political assassination thriller, the central character plans to have extensive plastic surgery, even on his fingerprints, to change his appearance and facilitate his disguise.[3] Detective novels are full of criminals who have had their faces or their fingerprints changed by plastic surgery.

Spy novels are even more colorful than detective stories. Dozens of spy novels have characters who undergo extensive plastic surgery to disguise their appearances or to make them resemble a certain person. The theme of an espionage agency grooming an agent to replace a key individual in the enemy camp is a common one. *The Spy Who Loved America*, by Charles Einstein, has a Soviet agent replacing a U. S. military officer. *The Kremlin Letter,* by Noel Behn, has an American espionage agency preparing an agent to operate inside Soviet Russia, and describes the measures considered in order to make him look the part.

In reality, there are few documented cases of plastic surgery used to change an agent's or fugitive's appearance. There are several reasons for this:

1. Some feats are impossible. A plastic surgeon cannot change fingerprints. Any surgeon can, by removing enough layers

of skin from the fingertips, obliterate fingerprints, and anyone who has the guts or desperation to undertake do-it-
yourself surgery can use a razor knife or caustics to do the
same. Given the state of the art, though, it's impossible to
generate new and different fingerprints. Worse, if too few
skin layers are removed, the old fingerprint pattern will
grow back.

2. As a strictly practical matter, anyone who has his fingerprints obliterated will attract an extraordinary amount of attention if ever fingerprinted for any reason. Police will
scrutinize very closely anyone they find without fingerprint
patterns on his fingertips. While the individual may succeed
in concealing his origins, he'll be under grave suspicion and
will surely face questions regarding why and how his fingerprints came to be obliterated.

3. The few real-life people who tried this didn't fare very well.
John Dillinger had plastic surgery on both his face and fingerprints, by an old doctor who had lost his license and was
reduced to treating gangsters for gunshot wounds. Yet, Dillinger still came to grief because he would not abandon his
old lifestyle. He still looked very much like his old self, and
he ended up shot to death after being snitched off to the FBI
by an informer. More, his scarred fingertips did not produce
fingerprint patterns, and this would have attracted notice if
he'd ever been arrested again.

4. Plastic surgery leaves scars, as does any surgery or injury.[4]
It's impossible to perform any surgery without leaving some
sort of scar, and although plastic surgeons are very careful
with both incising and suturing skin in order to leave minimal scars, the surgery still leaves traces. A competent plastic surgeon makes his incisions in the hairline, or in the
depth of a wrinkle, to make the scar blend in or to conceal it
altogether. The scar, however, is still there, and close examination will reveal it.

5. There may be problems in finding a plastic surgeon who will do the job. Plastic surgeons always want to know why a patient wants the surgery, and whether his expectations are realistic or not. Some refer applicants to a psychiatrist or psychologist to explore this question, and this can be troublesome.[5]

6. Although the modern period of plastic surgery began at about the turn of the century, much was, and still is, "vanity surgery," and thus has been somewhat disreputable in the eyes of other doctors oriented towards treating diseases and injuries.[6] The implications of this point are serious, as we'll see.

Plastic Surgeons

We can begin by looking at plastic surgeons, what sort of men (most are male, as we see from the Directory of Medical Specialists) they are, and what sort of skills they have. The popular image doctors foster is that of a skilled and altruistic healer. This is sometimes true, although many doctors are in the field mainly for the money. Plastic surgeons are a breed apart, as they specialize in vanity surgery, very different from the life-saving and healing arts. Dr. Reardon paints a very complimentary picture of plastic surgeons in his book,[7] but there's more to the story than that.

The basic fact is that plastic surgery, like all medicine, is a business, and the most successful practitioners are businessmen as well as surgeons. Some take a frankly mercantile approach to their trade, "marketing inferiority to women" in the search for more business.[8] Women are not the only categories contributing to the profitability of plastic surgery. These surgeons are perfectly willing to take advantage of ethnic minority members who want their noses re-shaped to look more Caucasian.[9] A significant part of plastic surgeons' business, therefore, comes from people who have been rendered dissatisfied with the way nature made them.

Business is good, because plastic surgery is costly. A point which bears very strongly on cost is that medical insurance doesn't cover vanity surgery.

The kind of plastic surgery covered by insurance usually involves the correction of disfigurement resulting from birth defects, injuries, or disease. Facial prosthesis, with synthetic features used to replace damaged ones, has expanded in recent years by the development of new materials, such as Silastic, which looks and feels like skin, and by acrylic eyeballs. These false features often look as good or better than the originals, although they cannot function like them. Surgeons attach some to the face with medical glue, while others are removable for cleaning. It's still necessary to use make-up to cover the margin where the prosthesis meets the face.

The purpose of a facial prosthesis is to match the original facial feature. A prosthesis wouldn't be very useful as a disguise, because your new face would look very similar to your old one. A conventional facial prosthesis is made only after the destruction of the original facial feature, and it's impractical for someone to sacrifice his vision, nose, or other feature for the sake of obtaining a prosthesis. In any case, this type of corrective surgery is not what we normally consider plastic surgery.

Traditionally, plastic surgery has been for the wealthy. Screen and TV stars, who feel that erasing the outward signs of advancing age is necessary for their careers, are very able to afford expensive plastic surgery. So are the jet-setters. Working people, though, have neither the money nor the inclination for such frivolities, and tend to believe that the less they see of doctors, the better.

Therefore, plastic surgery is a very remunerative occupation. A plastic surgeon doesn't have to accept a patient who may not be able to pay, and pay handsomely. Plastic surgeons tend to be "society" doctors, selecting their patients mainly for their affluence and ability to pay high fees.

Some health care professionals look down upon plastic surgeons, calling them "tits and butts" men. Presumably, this is because they do not practice life-saving surgery, limiting themselves only to safe operations. Plastic surgeons don't get into taxing brain or heart surgery, in which life hangs in the balance every moment. This is because plastic surgery is "elective" surgery, and plastic surgeons select patients carefully, avoiding those who present significant physical risks.

Apart from their wealth, what can we say about the skills of plastic surgeons? A doctor who calls himself a plastic surgeon or other specialist should have had a certain amount of training, but no law actually requires this. A license to practice medicine allows a doctor to practice any type of medicine he wishes.

Is Board Certification Important?

Each state has laws regulating medical practice, and generally they bar anyone who has not graduated from medical school, served an internship, and passed state-administered examinations from practicing medicine or surgery. As we've seen, a licensed doctor can practice in any area of medicine or surgery he wishes, but associations of medical specialists have set up procedures for training and accrediting specialists.

The official view of the American medical establishment is that any specialist should be "certified" by the specialty board involved. The official reason given is that certification ensures that the doctor is properly trained and qualified. On the surface, this sounds reasonable, but behind it is a hidden agenda. An important effect of limiting medical practice to those who pass the standards set up by other doctors is that it stifles competition.

The American Board of Plastic and Reconstructive Surgeons will certify a doctor who has had the required training and who passes a Board Examination, awarding him a certificate to hang on his wall. This represents the official and "politically correct" point of view.[10]

The *American Society of Plastic and Reconstructive Surgeons' Guide to Cosmetic Surgery* warns against those who do not have board certification.[11] This, too, is a corollary of the official point of view. The ASPRS is a professional organization, in fact very much like the American Medical Association, widely recognized as the most powerful union in the country.

With all that, what use is a medical specialty certificate? Realistically, it's very much like a driver's license. It merely means that the person demonstrated a certain level of skill at the time of the examination. It absolutely does not guarantee that the doctor has kept up with progress in his field. It also cannot guarantee that his skill hasn't declined.

One joke about doctors is that 50% of them graduated in the bottom half of their class. Another is that somewhere is the worst doctor in the United States, and that someone has an appointment with him tomorrow morning. These are just jokes, but they are based on facts. If you're considering plastic surgery, or any other type of medical care, you need to know a lot more than many doctors are willing to tell you.

Four Plastic Surgeons

To get a better idea of the variety of plastic surgeons in the field, let's look at a few, comparing their backgrounds and levels of skill. These are real people, known to the author, with names disguised to avoid lawsuits.

Dr. Craftsman practices in a large city in the Southwest, and has a good reputation among both his patients and his medical colleagues. He doesn't need to advertise, as word of mouth brings him all the patients he can handle. His patients speak of him as an artist as well as a surgeon, and he earns his acclaim by his careful work.

Dr. Carpenter is a slightly younger man, who operates his own clinic in a wealthy suburb of Dr. Craftsman's city. He is competent, but obviously has gone where the money is. He has a good reputation, and earns a good living.

Dr. Shoemaker is young, having been Board-certified only three years ago, and has established himself in a city to the south. His interest in money is blatant, and is obvious in the form he has every new patient complete. This form takes both sides of an 8½" x 11" sheet, devotes more space to questions about the patient's financial health than his physical health. At the time of the first edition of this book, Shoemaker was new in town, and could not charge the high fees that older, established plastic surgeons charge, but he's worked his way up the ladder as quickly as he could. Shoemaker was recently elected president of the state medical society.

Dr. Butcher is a professor in a medical school, and a perfect example of the principle that "Those who can, do; those who can't, teach." He has the prestige of his university position, and in fact is the one who taught Dr. Shoemaker, who describes Dr. Butcher as his "mentor." He is not very skilled, though, and his surgery shows this. The quality of Butcher's work resembles cheap and dirty emergency room surgery. He leaves out stitches, his patients have more than the usual complications, such as infections and hematomas, but these problems don't interfere with Dr. Butcher's opinion of himself.

Plastic Surgery: The Real Story

Let's take a look at the field of plastic surgery. We've already seen that plastic surgery is not life-saving surgery. Nobody dies of wrinkles or baldness. The main reason for plastic or "vanity" surgery is to change or improve appearance. Let's consider specific operations, avoiding the technical language that doctors love to use to baffle their patients.

Nose Job

This means re-shaping the nose, to correct or modify a hook, reduce its size, narrow the nostrils, or to correct a badly-set break. If the nose has a hook, the surgeon will go in through the nostrils and shave off part of the bone or cartilage causing the hook. In the case of a big nose, he'll remove part of the bone to reduce its size. When doing nose jobs, surgeons try to work from inside the nostrils to hide the scars. (See Figure 15-1.)

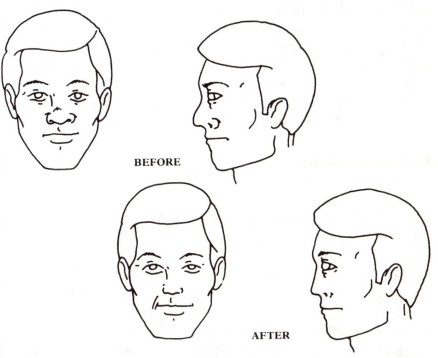

BEFORE

AFTER

Figure 15-1

A Nose Job.

To correct a badly set broken nose, the surgeon breaks it again and resets it properly.

Another type of nose job is to reconstruct a nose partly or completely destroyed from an injury. In one case, a person had slammed face-first into the dashboard of a car during an accident, flattening the nose. The surgeon used a section of rib to form the bone to give the nose its shape. Some people want their naturally small noses enlarged. Surgeons use both natural materials, such as bone and cartilage grafts, and synthetic materials, such as various types of silicones and plastics, to provide more bulk.

Ethnic minority members with wide or flat noses sometimes seek to have their nostrils narrowed. Re-shaping nostrils large and round enough to take a pair of .45-caliber cartridges requires removing wedges from the base of each nostril and stitching the edges together. This will result in a tapered look, more like Caucasian nostrils, and will leave only small scars under the nose.[12]

Costs of nose jobs vary widely. Surgeons' fees range from $1,500 to $5,000, according to a survey by the ASPRS.[13]

Hair Transplant

This is a technique to cover a bald spot by transplanting hair from another place. (See Figure 15-2.) Usually, this means that the person must be only partly bald, as there must be enough hair to furnish a transplant without totally denuding the donor site.

There are roughly two ways of doing a hair transplant: a strip graft, or using plugs. A strip graft is lifting a strip of hairy skin from a part of the scalp that isn't bald and transferring it to the bald spot. The plug technique is almost exactly the technique that landscapers use to re-sod a lawn: taking plugs from hairy patches and inserting them in evenly spaced rows in the bald area.

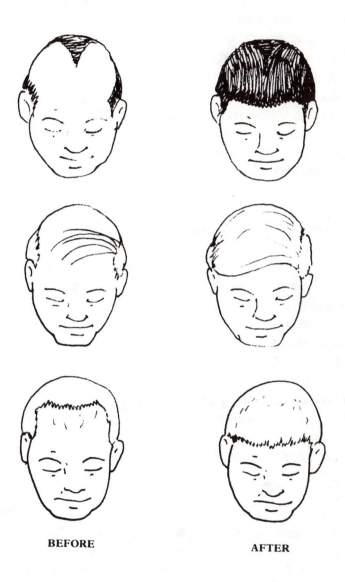

BEFORE   **AFTER**

Figure 15-2

Hair Transplant Surgery.

As with nose jobs, concealing the scars isn't much of a problem, as hair will cover them. The patient combs his hair to cover any scars, and combing and styling the hair after healing is complete is an important part of the process.

There are hair transplant clinics with surgeons specializing in such surgery. These are serious threats to plastic surgeons who do hair transplants, as the clinics advertise aggressively in the media. The official view of the ASPRS is that hair transplant clinic surgeons may not be certified specialists and that the patient may receive assembly-line treatment at the hands of someone who is inadequately trained.[14] However, this isn't necessarily the entire story.

Experience in other fields of surgery has shown conclusively that the quality of results increases with the number of operations done. Surgeons working in hospitals that do many open-heart operations each year have lower mortality rates than those doing only a few. Practice builds proficiency. A surgeon working in a busy hair transplant clinic, although lacking an "official" board certification, may well be more proficient than a conventional plastic surgeon who has the correct paperwork to adorn his office walls, but who does few procedures a year.

Costs of hair transplants, like those of other plastic surgery, vary widely. Depending on the procedures, the number of grafts, and the surgeon, cost can be anywhere from $750 to as much as $5,000, in 1992 prices.[15]

Eye-Lifts

Age and stress tend to cause bags under the eyes. These present a chronically tired appearance, although bags under the eyes are caused by fatty deposits under the lower eyelids, and not fatigue. If there's also a droopiness of the upper lids, it accentuates the fatigued effect.

To modify the upper lid, the surgeon removes a strip of skin from the upper lids, placing the cut along the line of the crease, making the scar less visible. To correct bagginess of the lower lid, he removes a strip of skin and part or all of the fat pads under the skin. (See Figure 15-3.) The scar line, immediately under the edge of the lid, is concealed by the eyelashes.

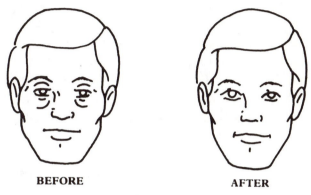

BEFORE   **AFTER**

Figure 15-3

Eyelift surgery— both upper and lower eyelids.

In some instances, there's a better cosmetic effect if the surgeon also removes a strip of skin immediately above the eyebrow, correcting what is called a "droopy brow" or "hound dog" appearance. The proper technique is to arrange the scar so that it's concealed by the eyebrow.

Surgeons' fees range from $1,000 to as much as $5,000, depending on the surgeon, locale, and whether the surgeon does the upper, lower, or all four lids.[16]

Ear Job

Many ear jobs are to correct congenital defects, as the ears don't droop much with age, although they may become hairier. Those considered congenital "defects" are often not defects at all, but only departures from the norm, as the ears work well despite their unusual appearance. For example, some people are concerned about their protruding ears, because ears that lay more or less flat against the head are the accepted look in our society. "Jug ears" can cause mental anguish, and they're also a conspicuous identifying feature.

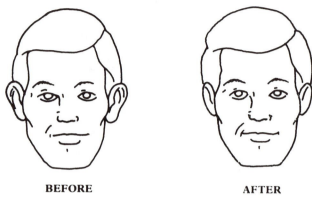

BEFORE   AFTER

Figure 15-4

Surgery to eliminate protruding ears.

To correct protruding ears, the surgeon makes a cut right behind the ear, exposing the cartilage of the ear and the bone next to it. He sews the cartilage to the bone, "pinning back" the ear, and removes any excess skin. The resulting scar will be at the juncture of the ear and skull, and inconspicuous. In many cases, hair will cover it. (See Figure 15-4.)

As with other plastic surgery, costs vary amazingly, from $1,000 to $4,000, according to the ASPRS.[17]

Chin Job

A receding chin, or "weak chin," is also open to correction by plastic surgery. (See Figure 15-5.) The operation usually leaves no visible scar because the surgeon makes his incision inside the lower lip and inserts an implant to re-shape the chin. The implant may be a piece of bone taken from another part of the body, or it may be silicone rubber. A variant of this technique is to cut the chin bone and slide the lower part forward or back, depending on the result needed.

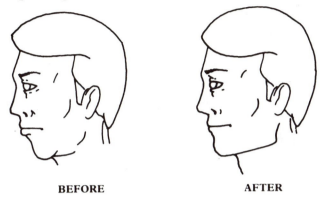

BEFORE   **AFTER**

Figure 15-5

Surgery to strengthen a weak chin.

An older technique was to make a half-moon incision under the chin, where it would be less visible from the front, but still noticeable from underneath. Working from inside the mouth is the preferred method, because the mucous membrane lining the mouth heals more quickly than exposed skin, and the scar remains concealed.

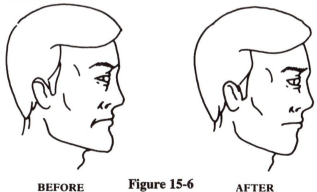

BEFORE   **Figure 15-6**   **AFTER**

Correcting a jutting chin with plastic surgery.

A plastic surgeon can also correct a protruding or jutting jaw. (See Figure 15-6.) The technique is to make the incision inside the mouth, then shave the jutting bone in front. Again, the scar remains concealed.

Both nose jobs and jaw jobs can change the profile greatly. While it remains impossible, given the state of the art, to change the shape of the skull, it's possible to modify the outer parts of the profile, and this can make a significant change in appearance. Costs vary with both the surgeon and the technique. Chin implants, according to an ASPRS survey, vary from $300 to over $2,000, while chin bone operations run from $600 to over $3,000.[18]

Face Lift

A face lift is merely a tightening up of sagging skin on the face, not a total re-shaping. It has nothing to do with congenital defects, repairing an injury, or correcting the shape of any part of the face. The face lift only alleviates the sagging and wrinkling of old age. (See Figure 15-7.)

Accordingly, the face lift is one of the most overrated practices in plastic surgery. Some think that it's a rejuvenation operation, but it's not. Skin inevitably changes with age, becoming thinner and less elastic, and no surgery can change this.[19]

One doctor, in a book promoting plastic surgery, points out that any alternative to a face lift has drawbacks.[20] Creams, massages, and other techniques are not permanent, according to him. However, a few pages further, he admits that a surgical face lift is not permanent, either,[21] in a section titled "The Second Face-Lift." Significantly, this book does not mention the costs of a face lift, or any other plastic surgery, except to state that plastic surgeons expect their patients to pay in advance.[22]

The operation itself, while simple in principle, requires careful work. The surgeon makes an incision at or near the hair line, undercuts the skin of the face, working through this incision. He then removes a strip of skin to take up the slack, and closes the incision.

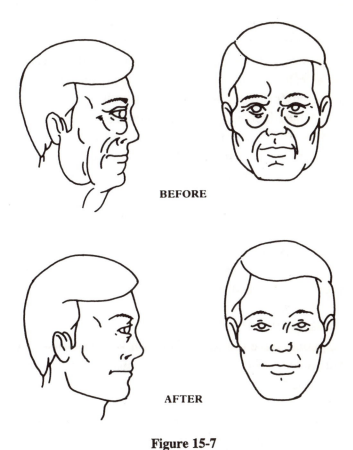

BEFORE

AFTER

Figure 15-7

Full Face Lift Surgery.

The face lift is in vogue among entertainers who have both the money and the need to maintain a youthful appearance. Unfortunately, some of these people fall victim to "youth doctors" who claim to be able to rejuvenate aging bodies by administering various drugs of dubious and unproven value.

Retarding the effects of aging is impossible. It's only possible to avoid bringing the effects on sooner. Visible effects arrive sooner with heavy smoking, drinking alcohol, use of some recreational drugs, poor diet, lack of exercise, and excessive exposure to sunlight. What used to be called "clean living" has a beneficial effect, because the person who avoids the use of tobacco and other drugs does not prematurely age his body.

Another hard fact is that aging occurs at different rates for different people. Both genetic make-up and lifestyle affect aging. Genetic make-up is irreversible, but lifestyle habits that age the skin, as we've seen, are open to modification. Genetic factors are very important, and some people just appear to age faster than others. For the person interested in living to a ripe old age, looking at his ancestors will reveal a lot. If his parents and grandparents look younger than most people their age, and if they're long-lived, apart from accident-induced death, his chances are better than if they'd sickened and died young.

Removing Blemishes

Some people have blemishes on their bodies, some of which are self-inflicted. Those who had themselves tattooed when young may regret it later, and try not to display the tattoo. Others have scars from injuries, or various types of cancerous and pre-cancerous growths on the skin, some of them in very visible places. Most of these are possible to remove, but we have to ask whether the cure may be worse than the disease.

As we've seen, all cuts in the skin leave scars, even carefully-done surgical incisions. Is it better to leave the blemish as it is, or to substitute a scar? In the case of a particularly unsightly blemish, such as a tattoo in a prominent place, the scar may be preferable. However, many tattoos are so deep that removal of the skin won't erase them. They'll remain visible, although somewhat faded. In some cases, a person might want to have such a prominent mark of recognition removed at all costs. In such instances, taking a chance with plastic surgery might be worthwhile, although the results are somewhat uncertain.

There are four basic ways to remove tattoos, and none is perfect. The oldest and simplest is simply cutting it out, removing as much skin as necessary, and leaving a scar or patch of white skin in place of the tattoo. A second way is abrasion, using a diamond burr or wire brush. This works mainly for lighter tattoos, in which the ink layer is shallow. Chemical peeling with trichloracetic acid is quick and cheap, but takes longer to heal. It leaves a mark, and works only on shallow tattoos. Laser removal is the fourth method, and still not very widely used. Lasers don't have as many side effects as do other methods of removal, but are more expensive.[23]

Removing scars and pits from smallpox and acne by skin planing, sanding, or chemical peeling often works. The technique is to remove the top skin layers. Skin planing uses a very sharp tool to remove the top skin to a depth adjustable by the surgeon. This is comparable to planing wood. The rough top layer comes off, leaving the smooth underlayer exposed.

Skin sanding, called "dermabrasion" by those who prefer fancy words to simple language, is also comparable to woodworking. The earlier techniques involved sanding the skin by hand, but today there is a motorized tool for this. The tool resembles a motorized disc sander, with a motor, chuck, and an abrasive disc, much like those available in hardware stores. The surgeon uses it to sand the skin, removing superficial blemishes.

Body Sculpture

Plastic surgeons are ambitious, and have experimented with reshaping the body for those patients who had a compelling need and the money to pay for it. Common types of body sculpture are correcting sagging breasts and buttocks (see Figures 15-8 and 15-9), hence the term, "tits and butts men."

Breasts and buttocks sag for several reasons. The most common reason is age, as muscle and skin lose their tone, causing breasts, buttocks, and the face to sag. Another cause is fat. Some of us are born chubby, and with society's emphasis on a slender appearance, some will take excess weight off by dieting. Large weight loss results in excess skin, which folds over and presents a baggy appearance.

The smallest group seeking body sculpture is composed of people who want excess fat surgically removed. It's possible to remove, with a couple of hours on the operating table, the fat that makes up a "beer belly," but this is an extreme measure and most surgeons will advise a patient to try dieting first.

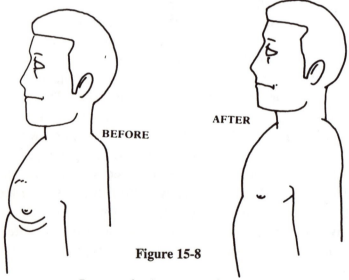

BEFORE

AFTER

Figure 15-8

Breast reduction surgery for men.

Some people have a fatty accumulation around each breast, and this can be embarrassing to males. This often happens in old age, but it can be bothersome to a young person of this body type. Some young people are grossly overweight in childhood, but make an effort to lose their extra fat during adolescence. This is a good time to diet on general principles, as normal growth takes up the slack of extra skin. In some cases, normal growth is not enough, and the teen-ager is left with sagging breasts or an abdominal "apron." If it bothers him enough, and if his family has the money, he may seek plastic surgery to eliminate this.

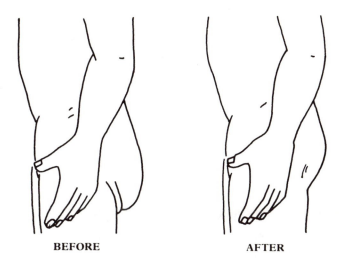

BEFORE   **AFTER**

Figure 15-9

Buttock reduction surgery can remove a sag, for a
more youthful and graceful appearance.

Breast and abdominal reduction, like other types of surgery, leave scars, but the plastic surgeon can minimize their prominence by carefully choosing where he cuts. For breast reductions, he'll most likely cut closely around the nipple, or make a half-moon incision where the underside of the breast meets the chest. For an abdominal reduction (see Figure 15-10), the resulting scar is usually at the groin and in the wrinkle where the abdominal skin meets the thighs.

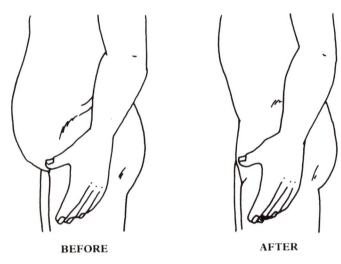

BEFORE   AFTER

Figure 15-10

Abdominal reduction surgery.

Liposuction is a new technique, originally developed in France, for removing fat by the use of a high-tech vacuum cleaner. The surgeon makes small incisions to allow insertion of the suction needle, which varies between one-eighth and three-eighths of an inch thick. He uses the needle to break up fat cell deposits and the vacuum sucks out the loose cells. The fee can be between $500 and $5,000 depending on the surgeon and the extent of the suctioning performed.[24]

Harelips
About one in 1,400 babies born have harelips as congenital defects.[25] This is the sort of defect that surgeons usually correct

soon after birth, and few people grow to adulthood with harelips. The main advantage of correcting a harelip early is that
skin heals more quickly in infancy and childhood. The resulting
scar has more time to heal and blend in with surrounding skin.
By the time the person reaches adulthood, there should be only
a barely visible hair-line scar. Unfortunately, only rarely is a
harelip scar totally unnoticeable, and most people born with
harelips have a visible irregularity despite corrective surgery.
Some men, especially if they're entertainers or other types of
public figures, may grow mustaches to conceal the scar.

Unusual Plastic Surgery Applications

"Sex-Change" or "Reassignment" Surgery

During the last thirty-five years, "sex-change" surgery has
attracted a lot of attention here and abroad. The term "sex
change" is inaccurate, because it's impossible to change anyone's sex by surgery. Gender depends not only on the superficial reproductive organs, but on sex glands and specialized internal organs, such as the uterus. There is no way now known to
create such organs if they're not already present.

Hermaphrodites, born with the glands of both sexes and
misshapen genitals, are another case. It's possible to remove the
glands of one gender, re-shape the external organs, and have
reasonably functioning sex as a result.

Transsexuals, such as a man who believes that he has a
woman's personality trapped in a man's body, can end up only
as ersatz members of the opposite sex. All a surgeon can do is
remove the external male organs, re-shape the skin to simulate
the vulva and vagina, and use hormone treatments to stimulate
the development of breasts and secondary sex characteristics.
The result is not a real woman, but a castrate. No such simu-
lated woman has yet borne a child, for obvious reasons.

The situation is similar in the even rarer instance of a woman who wants to be a man. The surgeon can remove the uterus and ovaries, and even construct an artificial penis, with an implant to produce erection, but cannot create a real man. With masculine hormones, the castrate may even be able to grow a beard, but will never be able to impregnate a woman because the castrate cannot produce sperm.

Sex-change surgery is impractical for disguise. Not only is it extreme, but the effect is strictly limited. A physical examination quickly reveals the counterfeit sex. Other sexual characteristics, such as body proportions, tend to remain the same. A man's body, with typically broad shoulders and narrow hips, contrasts sharply with the typical female body. The male voice is deeper, and sex simulation surgery doesn't affect this. Christine Jorgenson, the widely-publicized sex-change subject of the 1950s, still had a deep, masculine voice several years after her surgery.[26]

For disguise purposes, when the subject is not required to disrobe, it's possible to mimic the opposite sex with appropriate clothing and make-up. This is called "transvestitism," and a further discussion follows in *Appendix I.*

Height Reduction

This is rare, applied only when a person's extreme height is unbearable. About 25 years ago, a wire service story told of a young lady in Sweden who stood about 6'4" and who wanted to be shorter to improve her social life. The surgeon removed segments of her thigh bones, shortened the muscles to fit, thereby reducing her height by several inches. This, like "sex-change" surgery, is an extreme measure and the effect is even more limited. Consequently, a plastic surgeon would probably advise anyone seeking such surgery to have psychological counseling to enable him or her to live with the excess stature.

Foreskin Reconstruction

Some European Jewish males resorted to a little-known form of plastic surgery during the Nazi Era to conceal their ethnicity.[27] Judaism requires male circumcision in infancy, and in Europe this mark made them easily identifiable because European doctors don't think infant circumcision has any medical value. European males, except for religious minorities, are not circumcised, and circumcision is a definite religious identifier.

The Gestapo became aware that some Jews had obtained forged identity papers, and during their sweeps, took any suspicious males into a doorway or alley for a drop-your-pants inspection. Some Jews had plastic surgery to disguise or undo their circumcisions. Records of the era are sketchy, and as foreskin reconstruction was clandestine, nobody really knows how many people had surgical foreskin replacements or how successful they were.

The recent film, *Europa, Europa*, dealt directly with this theme, with the central character a Jewish teenager trying to escape discovery by concealing his circumcision. Although he did not seek plastic surgery, he tried unsuccessfully to tie the remaining shaft-skin over his glans with a piece of string.

Since World War II, interest in foreskin reconstruction has increased, sometimes to disguise ethnicity. Avri El-Ad, a blond and blue-eyed Israeli spy who was born in Austria under the name of Avraham Seidenberg, took this route when he assumed the persona of a German businessman to infiltrate Egypt. Using the name, "Paul Frank," he set himself up in Germany as a start to the deception. He serependitously encountered a German doctor with whom he became friendly, and one day told him that he was unhappy at having been circumcised. The doctor examined him, and stated that his penis had enough slack skin to stretch down to cover the head, and with his permission operated on him, narrowing the orifice so that the new hood would stay in place.[28]

Another Israeli agent, Wolfgang Lotz, had been born in Germany of a German father and a non-religious Jewish mother, and had not been circumcised when he was born in Germany. Also blond and blue-eyed, he was able to pass as a German businessman and infiltrate the Egyptian business community, gathering information for Israel.[29]

Today, the ethnic strife between Serbs and Muslims in Yugoslavia has led to a similar situation, and Serbs discover Muslim males by their circumcisions. No information has yet come out of Yugoslavia regarding any attempts to conceal religious origin by plastic circumcision reversal.

In the United States today, a growing segment of opinion views circumcision as useless mutilation, and some circumcised males have taken steps to be restored to their natural state.[30] Between 50 and 100 males have had plastic "uncircumcision" during the last 20 years, with varying degrees of success. Surgical foreskin reconstruction has proved impractical, being expensive and with a high rate of complications. By contrast, non-surgical restoration, by stretching the penile skin has caught on and today there are several thousand involved in this effort. We'll discuss foreskin restoration fully in a subsequent chapter.

Evaluation of Plastic Surgery

From this discussion, we can see that plastic surgery has limited benefits and is always expensive. One cost estimate was in *Plastic Surgery for Men*, by James Reardon. It's worth noting that the cheapest procedure in this 1981 book was listed at $500 for the surgeon's fee alone. 1992 prices quoted in *The American Society of Plastic and Reconstructive Surgeons' Guide to Cosmetic Surgery* are $3,000 for a nose job and $5,000 for a face lift.[31] You must also count the costs of hospitalization or an outpatient surgical facility. Indirect costs include time lost from work, travel, drugs, laboratory tests, and other incidentals which can total more than the surgeon's fee.

Anyone considering plastic surgery should be aware that plastic surgeons, like other doctors, expect payment without regard to the outcome. Plastic surgeons, especially, demand payment in advance. Unlike plumbers, auto mechanics, and other ethical tradesmen, doctors refuse to guarantee their work. In short, the risk is all yours.

What plastic surgery can and cannot do is critical. We've seen that it's impossible to rework one person to resemble another, especially if the difference in appearance is great. Using plastic surgery to impersonate another is usually impossible.

It's also impossible to make a radical change in the shape of the body or face. While surgical weight removal, such as liposuction, can take pounds off in a couple of hours on the operating table, dieting is much less costly, much less dangerous, and leaves no scars. It's impossible to change the shape of the skull, but changing the profile by modifying the nose or chin is workable. However, some surgical changes are not even permanent. Wrinkles and sags tend to return, and this brings up the question of cost-effectiveness.

Disguise is temporary. A wig, mustache, or other appliance put on with adhesive isn't permanent. It goes on and comes off quickly, allowing an appearance change in seconds or minutes. Plastic surgery, in many cases, is semi-permanent. In others, such as nose reduction, it is permanent.

The main value of plastic surgery, therefore, is to suppress or obliterate marks of distinction — features conspicuous because most people don't have them. This includes a harelip, a tattoo, a broken or misshapen nose, a jutting or weak chin, or other prominent blemish. In plain language, plastic surgery works best when used to make the patient look more ordinary, not when the patient wants to change an otherwise ordinary face or body.

When considering plastic surgery for disguise, it's important to recall that people tend to remember distinctive features, such as extreme height or corpulence, a squeaky voice, a nervous twitch, or an unusual facial feature. A description of "average height, coloring, build, weight, and face" is almost useless, because it fits so many people.

Summing up, plastic surgery's utility is limited. The person seeking to disguise himself can do at least as much with more conservative means, which are also cheaper and safer.

Notes

1. *The American Society of Plastic and Reconstructive Surgeons' Guide to Cosmetic Surgery*, Josleen Wilson, NY, Simon & Schuster, 1992, p. 13.
2. *Ibid.*, p. 15.
3. Brian O'Connor, *The One-Shot War*, NY, Ballantine Books, 1980. This is a typical shoot-em-up. The reference to plastic surgery makes it appear that it's as simple as having the teeth cleaned.
4. John A. McCurdy, Jr., M. D., F. A. C. S., *Cosmetic Facial Surgery*, NY, Frederick Fell Publishers, Inc., pp. 14, 52. There is even a chapter on scar revision, a technique to correct scars from injuries and previous plastic surgery.
5. *Ibid.*, p. 33. Part of the reason for this is the growing tendency among psychiatrists and psychologists to intrude into areas outside their fields. From treating the mentally ill, they've expanded their efforts so that today they "treat" people who are not mentally ill, but merely afflicted with normal problems of everyday life. Obviously, a "normal" person seeing a psychiatrist as an outpatient is more likely to be able to pay the exorbitant fees than a psychotic in a state hospital.

6. James J. Reardon, *Plastic Surgery for Men*, NY, Everest House, 1981, p. 17. Dr. Reardon's book is a very practical guide to what a man can expect from plastic surgery. Each discussion of a procedure has a section titled "What can go wrong," which shows a good deal of honesty on Dr. Reardon's part. This is in sharp contrast to the behavior of many other doctors, who push unneeded treatments and surgery on patients without adequately advising them of the risks.

7. *Ibid.*, p. 13. It's customary for doctors and other professionals to flatter themselves, but Dr. Reardon goes on to describe very seriously the possibilities and limitations of plastic surgery, and demonstrates that it cannot work miracles. Both his and Dr. McCurdy's book make efforts to correct some of the myths about plastic surgery.

8. *The American Society of Plastic and Reconstructive Surgeons' Guide to Cosmetic Surgery*, p. 16.

9. *Ibid.*, p. 85.

10. Reardon, p. 41. Wallpapering the office with diplomas and certificates is a common practice among medical specialists, as they know that people are impressed by fancy looking pieces of paper. For the patient, it's crucially important to look beyond the wallpaper at the doctor himself. The patient has the very difficult task of trying to evaluate the doctor's skill while knowing very little of the field, and the relationship involves a lot of blind trust.

11. *The American Society of Plastic and Reconstructive Surgeons' Guide to Cosmetic Surgery*, p. 16.

12. *Ibid.*, p. 87.

13. *Ibid.*, p. 97.

14. *Ibid.*, p. 208.

15. *Ibid.*, p. 209.

16. *Ibid.*, p. 176.

17. *Ibid.*, p. 112.

18. *Ibid.*, pp. 128-129.

19. *Cosmetic Facial Surgery*, p. 98. *Plastic Surgery For Men*, p. 152.

The effects of creeping age are definite and almost irreversible. Many people, concerned with the visible effects of advancing age, buy copious amounts of cosmetics promising a younger appearance. The cosmetics industry sells many millions of dollars of creams and lotions each year to people who use them to disguise or smooth aging skin.

Some women, in consternation over their fading good looks, apply make-up so heavily it seems to have been put on with a trowel. Others accept age more stoically and light-heartedly. One man, replying to someone's comment about his receding hair line, said: "The only trouble with going bald is that the lobotomy scar starts to show."

20. *Cosmetic Facial Surgery*, p. 109.
21. *Ibid.*, p. 123.
22. *Ibid.*, p. 17.
23. *Guide to Cosmetic Surgery*, pp. 159-161.
24. *Ibid.*, p. 278.
25. *Plastic Surgery for Men*, p. 206.
26. Personal observation by author, who met Christine Jorgenson by chance at a wedding reception.
27. Tushnet, L., "Uncircumcision," *Medical Times*, #93, 1965, pp. 588-593. Schneider, T., "Circumcision and Uncircumcision," *South African Medical Journal*, #50, 1976,pp. 556-558.
28. El-Ad, Avri, *Decline of Honor*, Chicago, Regnery, 1976. p. 114.
29. Blumberg, Stanley A., and Owens, Gwinn, *The Survival Factor,* NY, G. P. Putnam's Sons, 1981, p. 198. For the entire story of this extraordinary spy, see Lotz, Wolfgang, *The Champagne Spy*, NY, St. Martin's Press, 1972.

30. Bigelow, Jim, Ph. D., *The Joy of Uncircumcising*, Aptos, CA, Hourglass Book Publishing, 1992, Foreword by James L. Snyder, M.D., FACS.
31. *Guide to Cosmetic Surgery*, p. 68.

Chapter Sixteen

BODY-IMAGE

Whatever tangible and practical uses exist for disguise and other means of changing appearance, most who use these techniques seek to change what's come to be called "body image," rather than avoiding recognition. A man with a mustache covering a harelip scar, a beard hiding acne scars, or who combs his hair over a bald spot, does so to improve his appearance, not to become unrecognizable.

The term "body image" has a lot to do with what we call "self-image" — the way we see ourselves. We tend to see ourselves within a framework suggested or dictated by people around us, and by our culture in general. Some of the more important influences on the way we see ourselves are advertisements, TV, movies, and magazines.

Degrading the Self-Image

Years ago, before mass communication was developed, people obtained their ideas mainly from friends and acquaintances, real people whom they saw often. Today, unfortunately, many of our ideas about our self-images come from the mass media, based on entertainers and fictional characters. Two important facts strongly affect the picture:

1. Most programming on radio and TV is not concerned with real people, as news shows take up only a small part of the daily schedule. Most broadcast material is fiction, such as police shows, soap operas, and other dramas.
2. These fictionalized characters are not only unreal people; they are unlike most people in the real world. They're usually young, slender or athletic in build, attractive, well-spoken, and they have a sense of purpose.

Fantasy shows are attractive to us because they provide escape from the drab real world in which we live. The heroes are young, attractive, and they manage to solve their problems competently. For the most part, neither our lives nor ourselves are like these screen illusions. Obviously, the parts in screen and TV presentations are played by a group of unusual people — professional actors — and it's evident that actors are a group of especially attractive and articulate people chosen for exactly these qualities.

There's another category of fantasy with which we are bombarded by the media: advertisements. Produced specifically to sell a product or service, advertisements suggest that if we buy the product we'll be happier. Ads portray young and attractive people with cigarettes, bottles of soda pop, automobiles, and directly or indirectly promise that if we follow the examples shown and buy the products, we'll be as blissful as the smiling models.

Some ads are nagging in tone, highlighting real or imaginary defects which the products will supposedly allay. Perspiration, bad breath, gray hair, dry skin, and other physical qualities are the villains of these ads. The ads are designed to make us feel dissatisfied enough about ourselves and our appearances that we'll buy the products to enhance our self-esteem.

Americans, and people in some other industrialized countries, often suffer from degraded self-images. We're pressured toward conformity to a media image of unrealistically attractive and competent people. Media people are definitely not average, but present an unrealistic and unattainable ideal. We can't all be tall and slender, with regular and attractive faces. We also don't remain young forever.

Enhancing Appearance

Appearance is important to many people. They place great emphasis on seemingly minor details, such as using cosmetics and wearing the latest fashions in clothing. Some people even have their clothes tailored to minimize what they see as a physical defect. For example, a good tailor can cut a suit to conceal or disguise a flabby or pudgy body. Custom shoes have "lifts" to add an inch or two to the wearer's stature. Cosmetics hide pits and other blemishes in the skin. All of these devices fall into what we can call the "normal" range, because they're so common and easily obtainable.

Different people have different ideas regarding how they'd like their bodies to be. Understandably, many short people would prefer to be taller, and fat people would prefer being slender. Likewise, some thin people might like to be more muscular or athletic-looking. The measures people are willing to take, or at least consider, to conform to their ideas regarding body-image are sometimes extreme and surprising. This sometimes goes beyond physical attributes, depending on the group and the specific situation. Some body-image problems come from minority types trying to become like the White Anglo-Saxon Protestant majority.

Blacks have a difficult time of it, because most people who appear in the media are Caucasian. Some Blacks try to assume Caucasian physical characteristics, and buy preparations made to straighten kinky hair. Some wig companies make models with straight black hair, and their advertisements portray Blacks with Caucasian-appearing hair styles.[1]

Other ethnic groups have their own problems. Both Italians and Jews sometimes undergo plastic surgery and name changes to subdue or disguise their origins. The well-known "nose job" is for reducing or straightening a large or crooked nose. Name changes are common, with "Benedetto" turning into "Bennett" and "Weinstein" becoming "Winston."

These practices are not confined only to a few ethnic groups. Despite the long-promoted and "politically correct" ideal of the American "melting pot," where people of all nationalities, races, and religions live and work together harmoniously in a spirit of brotherhood, hard reality is quite different from the myth. Those who are Male, Caucasian, Anglo-Saxon, and Gentile, are often envied by those who are not.

Plastic surgery is often called "body-image surgery" because its purpose is most often to change appearance, not correct congenital or acquired defects. Most of the perceived defects "corrected" by plastic surgeons are not really mistakes of nature. A hare-lip is, but a big nose is merely a big nose. Likewise, sagging eyelids come from advancing age, and are perfectly natural, however displeasing to those who have them.

This is why we find people seeking physical changes for psychological reasons. A person buys a toupee, has a nose job, or wears custom clothing not for any reason of health or physical well-being, but to improve the way he feels about himself.

In certain instances, the effect sought directly contradicts nature. It's definitely not a birth defect to be born male or female, but there are a few people who feel that nature made a mistake in their cases. Some say that they're "women trapped in male bodies," while others feel the other way. This leads both to transvestitism, the fancy medical term for cross-dressing, and to "sex change" surgery.

Interestingly, most cross-dressers and gender change seekers are not psychotic. No successful sex-changers are, because they have to undergo psychiatric examination before being accepted for surgery and this disqualifies those obviously insane.

The Road to Change

Most people occasionally consider changing their body images. Many act upon these thoughts, changing hair styles or going on diets, but a few go to the extreme of plastic surgery. Anyone thinking about body-image change should do some soul-searching, with the effort proportional to the need, the expense, and the severity of the measure. It's important to keep the possible consequences in proportion to the perceived benefits.

Some steps are harmless, and almost trivial. Changing hair style is temporary. Anyone who decides that the change was a mistake can easily change it back the next day, although a crew cut or drastic shave can take weeks to undo. Cosmetics are usually harmless, and the risk is only the loss of the price paid for the product. Wigs, toupees, and clothing are somewhat more expensive, but again they cause no permanent change in the body.

The most serious steps involve surgery. Usually, this is not an impulsive decision. The person will have been thinking about it for years before making the final irrevocable decision to accept the rigors and expense of surgery as necessary evils, in order to feel better about himself.

Some types of body-image modification involve skin piercing which most people would not consider surgery. Piercing the nose or earlobes for rings is one example, and most who pierce ears and noses are not medical personnel. In larger cities, telephone classified pages have listings for "Ear Piercing."

A small subculture in the United States is into genital piercing. This results in placing a ring or a dumbbell like device called an "ampallang" into the glans, foreskin, or lips of the vulva. This is more serious, but still those who go in for genital piercing usually don't have it done by a doctor. Some want piercings for decorative purposes, while others say these devices enhance sexual pleasure. Anyone seeking genital piercing can often find someone to do it through a tattoo shop, or leather shop. Sex toy stores that sell rings and ampallangs can usually refer the buyer to someone who can install them.

Moderate Body-Image Changes

Most body-image efforts are not too rigorous, although they may seem so at times. Dieting is common among adult Americans, and anyone who has tried a diet knows the effort and self-discipline required. Body-building is another moderate effort, a slow, gradual process demanding will-power and time. The advantage of these methods is that, if the going becomes too tough at any point, the dieter can stop temporarily or permanently, an option lost by those who choose surgery.

All of these plans can be overdone, and there are slight dangers in both dieting and body-building. Some dieters go to the extreme of starving themselves, while some body-builders over-exert themselves and suffer muscle cramps and other physical problems. Yet, both have wide margins of safety and warning signs of impending danger, which allows most people to undertake them safely.

Psychological Counseling

Professional opinion to the contrary, psychological counseling is not necessary in most of these cases. Following the practice of American doctors to over-treat and over-prescribe, psychologists tend to feel that everyone, even those with minimal problems, need their services. Most people with problems have already discussed them with friends and relatives, and professional counseling can add little to this. Providing that the person concerned with body image does not have a mental disorder, professional counseling is unnecessary. In some instances, it can actually be harmful.

The professional counselor is in it for the money, and this affects both his viewpoint and his technique. Anyone turning to a relative or close friend for advice is not likely to find himself accepted or rejected depending on his ability to pay. A father or friend won't send a bill for his time, and will give the warmth usually lacking in professional relationships. There's a certain sincerity in family counseling that's hard to find or simulate in professional encounters.

Someone seeking help from a professional counselor may well find that the counselor has his mind on other things. If he's the last patient of the day, the counselor may be preoccupied with closing up shop and going home for dinner. Someone who runs out of money before running out of problems may find the relationship at an end, nevertheless. While it's unlikely that the counselor will be so rude as to show him the door, he may refer him to a public mental health office with a long waiting list, and the patient will have to start all over again with a new therapist.

Most people are more or less capable of leading their own lives, and do not end up in prisons or mental hospitals. Most people, most of the time, know what's good for them, and do not need professional intrusion. This is also true of body-image problems.

Motives, Risks, and Benefits

Those considering body-image alteration should give very careful thought to their motives. They should examine exactly why they want the change, and be sure in their own minds whether they're acting for their own internal reasons or because of peer pressure. Many people are conformists, wanting to be like everyone else, and it's at this point that they should assess the risks, costs, and benefits of body-image alteration.

On a simple level, it may be popular to dress in a certain style to fit in with the crowd. In certain occupations, such as the police and military, it's impossible to do otherwise. In others, it's hard to escape this pressure because of company policy or deep-rooted custom. An executive who normally wears a three-piece suit would face a reprimand if he showed up in jeans and a sweatshirt.

Some young people feel pressured to have tattoos, if they're members of the armed forces or of certain social groups. For some, wearing a tattoo means being a big man. This is more serious than clothing fads, because unlike clothing, a tattoo doesn't come off at the end of the day. It's designed to be a mark for life, and can become a stigma in later years. It's often possible to have a tattoo removed by surgery, at some risk, but the results are uncertain because of scarring.

Anyone considering changing body-image should, like a person contemplating other kinds of lifestyle changes, think carefully about costs and benefits. People change jobs and even occupations for more money, a reason which is tangible and clear-cut. Reasons for body-image change are not often as clear. They're intangible, tied in with the reactions of other people and with the person's feelings about himself.

It may be justifiable to change to conform to other people's expectations or demands, if the rewards justify the changes. Following a company dress code is justifiable if the job pays adequately or is otherwise satisfying. Conforming to the standards of a crowd or social group is less easy to justify in terms of rewards. What is social acceptance worth? It's impossible to value it in money.

Another practical aspect of conforming to crowd values is that the circle of friends and associates changes with time. Today's needs become obsolete tomorrow. If the change is permanent, the person may be laden with it long after the need has disappeared. In the cold afterlight of the day after tomorrow, he or she may feel that it wasn't worthwhile.

Internal reasons don't change as radically or as often as do social circles. Therefore, someone changing his body image for his own reasons will probably continue to enjoy the results.

Often, motives are mixed. There will be both internal and external reasons for change, and some of the external reasons may be very compelling. A grossly overweight person has good reason for dissatisfaction with his body image, detesting his appearance, and at the same time acutely aware that his obesity degrades his attractiveness to the opposite sex. He will almost surely be aware of the health risks of severe obesity. This provides a complex of reasons to try to change, and may give him the motivation to begin and maintain a diet.

The obese person realizes that if he sheds his excess weight, he'll look better, feel better about himself, and probably will live longer. Dieting isn't easy, as it taxes the person's will power, but it's not terribly risky nor does it involve an irrevocable commitment as do some more serious steps. Once started on a diet, the rewards begin to come. There's a satisfaction at seeing the weight melt off, and a gradual improvement in self-confidence as his body image approaches his expectations.

The intangible, but still very real, effects of changing body-image are the satisfaction and self-confidence that come with it. In severe instances, such as facial disfigurements, it means the shedding of self-consciousness and hang-ups.

Changing body-image is a decision that each person must make for himself. Other people's opinions, while important, are secondary, as he is the one who will have to live with the effects long after the others are gone.

Notes

1. Afro World Hair Company brochure.
    7262 Natural Bridge Road
    St. Louis, MO 63121

Chapter Seventeen

FORESKIN RESTORATION

Routine infant circumcision is a useless mutilation, but circumcision advocates have "pushed" this surgery for many reasons. Some claim circumcision prevents cancer, sexually-transmitted disease, and other problems. European males, intact except for a few religious minorities, have lower rates of STD and AIDS than Americans. Others state that circumcision makes the boy like his circumcised father, or trimmed playmates, advocating a type of surgical conformism that would produce loud protests if done to females. In fact, the influx of Moslems to this country has begun to raise female circumcision as a women's rights issue. Some circumcised males who are aware of this prefer to be natural again, now seeing it as a men's rights issue.

These males feel that men, like women, have a right to their own bodies. When the topic appears on a radio or TV show, as it did on Donahue several years ago, thousands of letters and phone calls come in to support groups.[1] An important reason is that despite the myth that infant circumcision is virtually risk-free, many are poorly done, and lead to complications.[2] Adult males seeking foreskin restoration information reported a 32.5% rate of physical complications. An earlier study of circumcised infants, by a physician, involved physical examinations and follow-up to age 6 months, which makes it the most definite of all studies. This doctor found a 24% rate of serious complications.[3] It's clear that infant circumcision is not benign or risk-free. However, males have sought foreskin restoration for other, more fundamental reasons.

Reasons For Restoring the Foreskin

Cosmetic — Some prefer the look of the natural penis.

Psychological — Being "all there" and natural provides more self-confidence and enhances the male's self-image.

Sensitivity — Removing the foreskin destroys its mucous membrane lining, containing sensitive nerve endings that enhance sexual pleasure. The exposed penis-head dries out, rubs against clothing, and loses sensitivity. Sometimes, the sensitive frenulum is removed along with the foreskin. Although the frenulum and the foreskin lining can't be replaced, recovering the head causes it to become soft and moist again, and more sensitive.

Sexual Manipulation — The foreskin is a natural stimulator, either through stroking back and forth during masturbation or foreplay, or by gliding action during intercourse, as a natural "tickler."

What to Expect From Restoration

The new foreskin may be quite satisfactory cosmetically, but amputated nerve endings are gone forever. A missing frenulum can't be replaced.

Almost everyone who has had his foreskin restored has had an increase in the sensitivity of the head, after a few weeks or months. Usually, this enhances sexual pleasure. The age at which the foreskin was amputated affects sensitivity. Those cut after infancy regain the most. The earlier the foreskin was amputated, the longer the head has been exposed and dry, rubbing against clothing. If the foreskin is removed at birth, the tender head of the penis is exposed to the irritation of wet diapers. At birth, the foreskin adheres to the head of the penis, not separating naturally until much later. Circumcision involves separating it forcibly with an instrument, which causes damage to the surface of the head, leaving pits that remain throughout life.

Removing the frenulum, the "G-string," under the head, results in the loss of a very sensitive part of the penis. Doctors rush through infant circumcisions, usually not even using anesthesia, and more damage than necessary occurs.

Before Starting

The function of the foreskin is to protect the tender head. Most foreskins cover the head fully and retract with erection to expose the head to sexual stimulation. Nature provides variations, though.

Foreskin length is genetic, as are penis length and the size of the head. Most foreskins cover the head, but some cover it only halfway. The foreskin is usually long and tight at birth, but loosens during childhood. The penis may outgrow its foreskin, so that some men have part of the glans exposed, even when limp. In erection, the penis swells and the head slides out of its protective covering. Some foreskins, however, are long enough to cover the head even during erection. In such instances, the foreskin retracts from thrusting or is pushed back manually.

Well over 80% of natural males have foreskins that partly or completely cover the head, according to one survey. Very few have the head completely exposed, and very few have such long and tight foreskins that they can't retract them.

Most restoration-seekers want the head fully covered. Some want an overhang beyond the tip, because they find it erotic. A tiny proportion want only more slack in the shaft-skin, covering only the rim at most.

Some males feel that nature short-changed them in genital size. Some, while satisfied with the length of the penis, wish that they had more foreskin. Not surprisingly, some uncircumcised males have sought information on how to lengthen their foreskins.

Head sensitivity varies, and this has a lot to do with the foreskin length desired. Some want the head fully covered, for maximum protection and return of sensitivity. Others find that friction from clothing or drying out from constant exposure irritates the head, and they too want full coverage.

Some consider esthetics important, and want a tapering overhang, in the manner of classic Greek statues. This can be a problem, because even many natural foreskins don't have this taper. Reducing the orifice of a gaping foreskin requires surgery, taking a "tuck" out of the tip. This carries the usual surgical risk, and may not give the desired result.

Yet others rank sexual manipulation as most important, and a long foreskin contributes to the length of the stroke in foreplay and masturbation. The really ambitious ones want two or three inches of overhang. The wide disagreement on how long the foreskin should be means that each must decide for himself, because there is no "proper" length.

Surgical Foreskin Restoration

There are two basic ways of restoring the foreskin, surgical and non-surgical. Surgical methods use a skin graft to cover the penis head. Some methods require only one operation, but others require more. Multi-stage procedures do not provide better results, but are more expensive.

The experience of several years and well over a dozen patients has shown that surgical foreskin restoration has severe risks of complications. These complications are beyond the usual surgical side effects such as post-operative pain, etc. Even the few totally satisfied with the results of surgery have had complications.

Between 50 and 100 males have had such surgery during the last 20 years. Some published their experiences. At least eight surgeons were involved. Their experiences demonstrate that surgical restoration has many disadvantages:

A. Few surgeons do foreskin reconstruction, and seeking one is an ordeal, often requiring travel to another city. Some doctors ridicule the patient or show hostility, and others tell the patient he needs a psychiatrist. Some plastic surgeons insist on a psychiatric examination, which can add hundreds of dollars to the total cost, and is irritating to patients who know no mental exam was required before their circumcisions. Those who consented to psychiatric examination submitted because it was required, not because they felt that it would help them.

B. Skin grafts involve cutting the nerve supply of transplanted skin, which leaves the new graft without sensation.

C. Results are uncertain. Some patients find the results satisfactory, but others do not. An important reason is that the process is under total control of the surgeon, not the patient, and the surgeon may make the graft too long, too short, too tight, etc. In this regard, many plastic surgeons insist on non-refundable advance payment, because they often do not satisfy the patient.

D. The graft usually does not match the color or texture of the shaft skin, resulting in a "two-tone" appearance that some find objectionable. This is particularly true of scrotal grafts, and the transplant is wrinkled and hairy.

E. With a scrotal graft, the new skin tends to contract with the slightest chill, as when undressing in a cool room or stepping from the shower. This makes it difficult to retract, interfering with urination. This effect is permanent.

F. Cost of surgery usually runs between five and twelve thousand dollars or more, not always covered by medical insurance. With cost of travel, and of psychiatric examination, the total is more than most can pay. Some surgeons want payment in advance, and fees for this surgery have, over the last fifteen years, risen faster than inflation.

G. There's a large risk of complications, which surgeons are usually not eager to discuss. The more involved procedures carry the greater risks, such as infections, hematomas, and sloughing off of the transplant. One patient underwent 13 operations which failed. Other complications can be mild or severe, and sometimes very painful. Well over 50% of surgical restorations result in complications.

H. The patient is sexually incapacitated during the recovery period, which takes weeks or months.

I. Surgery always leaves scars, which vary with the skill of the surgeon. They may be barely visible, or prominent and ugly.

J. Appointments must usually be made well in advance, requiring the patient to arrange for absence from work. There have been instances of patients arriving to find the surgeon out of town. In one case, the delay was three days before he could see the surgeon. In another, eleven days' delay caused the patient great inconvenience.

Anyone considering surgery should note that surgeons usually gloss over the risks in discussions with potential patients. Inspection of letters sent to inquirers by several of these surgeons showed that they either don't mention any risks or dismiss them with a few bland words. This has led to several people consenting to surgery which they later regretted.

The individual's willingness to take risks for his goal are often decisive. Many are willing to pay any price (medical insurance often doesn't cover this) and run any risks. They are often willing to settle for mediocre or plainly bad results. The high cost of plastic surgery often comes to more than just money.

Non-surgical Methods

These involve stretching the shaft-skin to cover the head of the penis, using tape to hold it in place. The principle isn't new. Primitive tribes have used various methods to stretch lips, earlobes, etc., for tribal identification or as marks of beauty. Documentation has appeared in *National Geographic*, and *Ripley's Believe It Or Not.*

This method takes time, requires much personal effort and emotional fortitude, as do dieting and body-building. Anyone who uses the stretching method must be well-motivated, persistent, and not easily discouraged, as results come slowly.

There are advantages to the non-surgical method. The cost is low, because the candidate buys tape and some other materials locally. There's no scarring, and no mismatched tissue on the penis. There is no cutting of the nerve supply, and little risk. This is why most men seeking restoration have chosen non-surgical methods over surgery.

Stretching goes in three stages: INITIAL, EQUILIBRIUM, AND EXTENSION. It's best to do this under medical supervision.

Seeking a trustworthy doctor involves the risk of being ridiculed and insulted, but with enough persistence, it's possible to find a sympathetic doctor. As a rule, younger doctors are more likely to have modern ideas.

The Initial Stage

First, measure the penis limp, along the top, from base to tip. Next, measure how far you can pull the skin up over the head, during erection, with both light finger pressure and with as much force as you can without pain. Record these measurements, as they'll be a guide to your progress. Measurements during erection will be the best guide because the size of the limp penis varies greatly.

The Tape Strap

After a hot bath, to make the skin soft and loose, pull it as far over the head as it will go, without pain. Use a piece of tape to strap it in place, running the tape from side to side, not top to bottom. Taping to the side will make it easier to urinate with the tape in place. For some people, it will be necessary to sit down to urinate.

One person reported success using "ELASTOPLAST" fingertip bandages for basic strapping. This flexible material adapts well to the contours of the penis. The four long flaps are the right length for correct strapping. One type is manufactured by Duke Laboratories, and found in drugstores. Cut or punch a hole in the center to allow urination. Position the hole over the meatus.

If you were cut tightly, squeeze the blood out of the glans before putting on the tape. That will enable you to get more skin taped up. When the blood returns to the glans, it will create tension to stretch the skin.

In squeezing, it's important to give one long and firm squeeze, not a series of short ones. Squeezing the glans stimulates the bulbocavernal reflex, producing throbs in the root of the penis, and causing erection. Erection impedes taping.

Problems With Tape

Over twenty percent of those using tape have problems with it. Some people have sensitive skins, and others are allergic to it. Many types of tape have worked for this, but it's best to start with the gentlest and least likely to irritate, such as 3M Micropore or J&J Dermicel, non-allergenic paper tapes. If these are not adhesive enough, and you have no rash or other reaction, you can use something stronger, such as white cloth surgical tape. Other types of tape which some have used are masking and electrician's tape, and various types of transparent and flesh-colored first-aid tapes. The usual width for best results is ½", but you can use whatever is most comfortable. You must find the tape that's best for you. White cloth surgical tape holds best, but is hardest to remove. Removing the tape too often can cause skin irritation in this sensitive area. Some make the mistake of removing the tape each time they urinate. Cellophane tape, with its sharp edges, cuts into the skin. Taping too tightly has also caused problems.

If you need more adhesion from the tape you use, you can paint the skin with tincture of benzoin, also known as "Friar's Balsam," sold in drugstores. This coats the skin with a tacky layer which increases the sticking power of the tape.

It's essential to avoid pain, nature's way of telling you that you're hurting yourself. Pain from taping too tightly suggests that you're causing slight internal tears in the skin, which will scar and contract as they heal, slowing progress. Some find that erection causes the tape to come off. Others complain that erections with the tape in place are painful. If erection causes pain, remove the tape immediately.

In those who were cut very tightly, there won't at first be enough skin to cover the head completely when taping. In this case, it's important not to let the tape strap touch and stick to the head, as removal will hurt. A square of tape face to face with the strap, where it contacts the head, will prevent this. Another way is to put a dab of talc on the tape where it contacts the head. Yet another way is to coat the front of the head lightly with Vaseline, being careful not to get any on the shaft-skin. It's also important that the skin of the penis be clean and free from sweat and body oils, which impede the tape's adhesion.

Handling the penis while taping may cause an erection, which makes taping more difficult. An ice pack, masturbating, or just waiting will make the erection go down.

You'll notice that with the tape on, the penis will be foreshortened and that the gentle tension on the skin from the pressure of the head will cause the skin to stretch. Erections also help stretching, if they're not painful.

For full effect, it's best to wear boxer shorts that let the penis hang, as its weight helps the stretching effect. Jockey shorts confine the penis, and interfere with stretching.

Avoid removing the tape too often. Taking it off for sex or urination can cause irritation or tear the skin. One way to allow urination with a tape strap is to use a paper punch to make a hole in the center for urine.

How Long Does Restoration Take?

The size of the penis, the length of the head, and the amount of skin cut off all affect the time needed to get results. Generally, those who were not cut tightly take less time than those who were. A lot of slack provides a head start. Your goal is also important. If you just want enough skin to cover the head with the penis limp, it will take less time than if you want skin for overhang, or to cover the head during erection.

In stretching, some have attained full coverage in four months. Others have taken longer. Some have been at it for three years and still don't have what they want. The most important factor is the effort and persistence you put into it.

Results

Usually, the first result noticed is a change in the color and texture of the head of the penis, which becomes pink and moist from being constantly covered, and regains sensitivity. This happens within a few weeks.

You'll notice that the skin will stretch noticeably for a week or so, then progress will stop for a few days. These periods of "rest" are inherent in the process, and we know of no way to overcome this stop-and-go pattern. This leads to elation when results are visible, and despair when progress stops. A similar effect exists with dieting and body-building. Persistence and coping with discouragement are vital to success. A person on a diet who gives up when he stops seeing daily weight loss will fail. Only long-term results count.

Stretching

It's important to wear the tape constantly. Only constant, gentle tension will stretch the skin permanently. It's a mistake to try to speed up the process by sudden, sharp pulls. As discussed before, this can cause internal scars. One man who did this tore the skin and caused bleeding. Although it may seem a waste of time to keep the tape on when nothing seems to be happening, it's important to keep the head covered to regain and maintain the sensitivity.

You can remove the tape for washing and for sex, but if you don't wear it almost 24 hours a day, progress will be much slower. If your schedule doesn't permit you to keep the tape on at least eight hours a day, it's not worth even starting.

Recording Progress

Keep a written record of your progress and, if you can, take photographs every month. It gives a psychological boost to have tangible proof of your progress as you go.

The Tape Ring

Once the skin has stretched somewhat, or if you were not cut tightly, you can use the tape ring. Stretch the skin out beyond the head and wrap a length of ½" tape around it to form a ring tightly enough to hold it in place but not so tightly as to interfere with urination or blood circulation. As a rule, if urine will pass, blood circulation will be unobstructed. Too loose a ring may slip behind the head and cause constriction, especially during erection. If this happens, remove the tape at once and use a smaller ring.

Some have had success using an "O-Ring" instead of a tape ring. An "O-Ring" is a rubber ring, usually used as a sealing ring, and obtainable in hardware stores. They come in different diameters, and the ones most useful range between ½" and ¾" in diameter. In choosing the ring size, it's important to find a size that holds the skin without impeding circulation to the skin forward of it.

Penile Hygiene

It's not necessary to wash the penis daily, because it doesn't get very dirty. Penile cleanliness has been over-emphasized for years, and many circumcisions were done because parents worried unduly about keeping their son's penis clean.

After several days or weeks, you may notice a whitish secretion collecting under the skin. This is smegma, cast off surface skin cells, and is perfectly normal. It acts as a lubricant, and the only reason for washing it off is if the odor is offensive.

Do not forcibly remove the tape for washing. Let it loosen by itself, from sweat and skin oil. When you can remove it without pain, you can wash. Washing requires only water, though some use mild soap. Some uncircumcised males have caused irritation by using strong soap on the sensitive skin of the penis.

You may want to remove the tape before it's loosened by itself, for sex. This may be irritating, and you'll have to judge the situation for yourself.

If you find it difficult to get rid of the last drops of urine after urination, a pad of toilet paper worn inside the shorts will absorb it. Once you're restored, slip the foreskin back to clear the hole when urinating.

Psychological Results

Usually, those who begin self-restoration experience a lift from contacting support groups, such as those listed at the end of this chapter, deriving benefit from contacting people sympathetic to their needs. There's also a lift provided by the realization that their circumcision mutilation need not be permanent, that they can do something about it, and regain control over this aspect of their lives.

You should realize that, while being intact again is very satisfying and will improve your self-image, it will not solve all of life's problems. A foreskin will not guarantee success in sex or anything else, just as dieting will not assure happiness.

Well over half of those circumcised in infancy or childhood blame their parents for this. Unfortunately, parents often simply follow the doctor's advice.

Some people blame circumcision for many unrelated problems that they have. After restoration, they may be unpleasantly surprised to find that they still have these problems.

Realistically, there are more problems in life than being circumcised, and being natural again is only a start towards solving them. The boost in self-confidence which accompanies being whole again is important, but realistic expectations will avoid disappointment later. The results of self-restoration, while better than any other method, are still not perfect and not quite a duplicate of the natural, uncut penis.

It's also important not to fool yourself about progress. It goes slowly, and it's easy to convince yourself that you're going faster than you really are, leading to later disappointment.

Partner Support

You should be doing this for yourself, not at the urging of a partner or wife, or because of peer pressure. There have been several instances of men who were circumcised as adults at the insistence of a wife or partner, and regretted it later. It can work the same way with restoration. If you feel comfortable circumcised, don't seek restoration simply because another person wants you to. It's equally important that your wife or lover not be strongly opposed to your wish to be natural again. There have been at least two instances of men who ran into strong opposition from their wives, which impeded their efforts.

Experimentation

Many restoration candidates devise other methods of stretching than those listed here. For those who want to experiment, it's important to avoid using anything with sharp edges, and to avoid blocking blood circulation to the skin. Any method which puts tension on the penile skin will work, as long as it does no harm.

Do not use clamps, elastic, heavy weights, or any other device or material that may cause injury, in an effort to speed up the process. In particular, don't risk cutting off the blood supply in the skin, as this can lead to serious consequences.

There are three ways to tell if the blood supply is being restricted:

1. Pain. This means the tape is too tight. Loosen it.
2. Color change. The skin turns blue and feels cold.
3. Test for constriction by pressing your finger on the skin hard for about fifteen seconds. Remove your finger. The spot where you pressed will be lighter in color. If it does not return to normal color within six to twelve seconds, the blood flow is impaired. Loosen the tape.

Most of the techniques and innovations described here have come from those experienced in stretching methods, who tend to be very inventive in devising variations of the basic methods. Some devise appliances that increase the rate of stretch. In doing so, it's critically important to avoid using anything with a sharp edge that will press into the skin. Even a ninety-degree angle, unless it's softened or rounded, can cause irritation, cutting, and bleeding. Keep in mind that anything sharp, even if not a knife-edge, will cut into the skin if pressed against it for hours or days.

If there's pain, stop at once! Don't try to tough it out. You're doing something wrong. While strong tension on the skin will make it stretch faster, it should not be so strong as to cause pain.

People vary in sensitivity to pain. This is why each must find his own level in taping, especially when experimenting with something not in the instructions, or without medical supervision.

Stretch marks occasionally occur. A light coat of cocoa butter, or other skin softener, applied after the tape is in place, will help. If you apply it before taping, it will keep the tape from sticking.

The Next Stages

As you progress, you'll approach the point of *EQUILIBRIUM*, where the length of the penis with the tape applied equals the original measurement without the tape. This is about as far as the skin will stretch with the initial methods. Next comes the *EXTENSION* stage, which will provide some overhang. This will help the orifice to narrow and keep the skin covering the head naturally. Without overhang, the new foreskin will tend to retract too easily.

Don't try to push the process along prematurely, as using advanced methods requires a certain amount of skin, without which it will be frustrating. There are, however, advanced stretching techniques.

Some males use a small rubber ball under the skin to get more stretch. The bulk of the ball, added to the bulk of the glans, helps put more tension on the shaft-skin when it's taped over it.

Another method reported is to use a plastic artificial penis, insert the penis inside, and tape the skin over the head of the artificial one. Being a sex toy, this device is more expensive than others.

Another individual uses a product called "Friendly Plastic," which is plastic that melts at about 140 F., to form an insert to hold his glans back while he tapes the skin up over it. This device looks like a thick golf tee, and is hand-molded to fit over the glans. The stem is about ¾" thick. Total length varies from two to four inches, depending on individual preference. You can obtain Friendly Plastic in an art store, and it costs about five dollars for a 4.4 oz. can, enough to make at least three devices. The manufacturer's address, as listed on the package and advertising literature, is: Friendly Plastic, Ltd., Boulder, CO.

Another variation on this theme is to get wide base nipples for disposable baby bottles. One brand is "Evenflo," and a blister pack of two sells for $1.19. Cut the flange off cleanly. Make sure to round the edges to avoid getting cuts or painful pressure. Cut a hole in the end for urination, place over the glans, and tape the skin in place. Use a paperclip through holes pierced in the end to hang a four-ounce weight, for tension. In preparing this device, be very careful regarding sharp edges, as even soft plastic can cut if pressed into the skin for long. These devices are very cost-effective.

Another reported using a sun lamp, which he said made the shaft-skin more flexible. He covered the head of the penis while using the sun lamp, as this is very sensitive mucus membrane and vulnerable to sunburn. It's important to cover right down to the scar line, as tissue in front of the scar is left-over mucus membrane from the inner lining, and also vulnerable. One device is a 35mm plastic film canister. Protection is essential, because sunburn can cause further loss of sensitivity.

Another stretching technique is using a balloon. For this, you tape the hood shut over the stem of a deflated balloon, which you have inserted underneath the skin. Use a non-oily lubricant, such as K-Y, and inflate the balloon with compressed air or CO_2. A can of "DUST-OFF" will work fine. This will stretch the skin a lot. The individual who devised this also advised that it works very well by inflating the balloon with hot water.

Yet another reported using a soft foam plastic ball under the skin, ahead of the glans, to get more stretch. Taping the skin forward over the plastic foam exerts more tension.

Some have used a weight to extend the shaft-skin. One good suggestion is to insert a large ball bearing under the skin and tape the skin over it. The ball bearing should be at least one inch in diameter to have enough weight to work well. The highly polished surface will not scratch or gouge the sensitive tissue.

Penile sensitivity is important, and increases as the head becomes moist again. However, a prescription ointment made by Ortho Pharmaceuticals is called "Retin-A." A little bit applied to the head of the penis appears to make the outer layer of dead cells slough off. To use, you apply a small amount, about the size of a pea, and massage it in thoroughly. The penis must be very clean before starting, to make sure that no layer of oil or other secretions acts as a barrier. In a few days, you will see small patches of cells sloughing off. You should be very cautious in applying this, and not assume that just because some is good, more will be better.

Retin-A is available by prescription only, and this means that you have to get a doctor's supervision. Surely you can find a doctor who will support you in what you're doing.

There are a couple of over-the-counter creams available, such as "Retinol," which probably contain the same active ingredient in a lower concentration.

A commercial product offered for foreskin restoration is the set of appliances called "Foreskin Restoration Cones," sold in sets of three different lengths. These produce more tension on the new hood.

Overall, these cones are well-designed and well-made. Unless the user does something stupid, the risk of injury is slight. The best feature of the design is how they avoid sharp 90-degree edges. The next best feature is the three progressive sizes.

One problem is that, although each cone has a hole drilled to allow urination, this is chancy because the hole is very difficult to align perfectly with the meatus. Another problem is that usually the diameter of the urethra is larger than the diameter of the tunnel provided.

The narrow channel causes back-pressure, and urine tends to flow out from under the cone and leak out through the outside of the cone and the tube of skin. In any event, it's really hard to get all the urine out. Some always remains, to leak out later. A wad of facial tissues helps. One user wears a condom with a cotton ball in the end. This is better than trying to remove the tape.

Finally, there is a chamfer, or countersink at the inside end of the urine tunnel. This is to allow for slight misalignment between the meatus and the tunnel, and avoids 90-degree edges which can cut the glans. Actually, some of the glans tissue flows up into this countersink and produces a little nipple protruding from the front of the glans where it flowed into the chamfer. This makes it imperative never to leave the cone on for several days straight, because with prolonged pressure, the nipple may become permanent.

It's important not to put the cone on too tightly during the first few days. It's also important to see how it works on each individual penis, as the same taping technique and particularly the same degree of tightness cannot work the same way for everyone.

The cones, with instruction sheet, are available from:

Second Skin
1335 Kentucky Street #5
New Orleans, LA 70117
Attn: Jay Borne
Cost is $39.00, post-paid.

Foreskin Restoration Support Groups

NOCIRC
PO Box 2512
San Anselmo, CA 94979-2512
Phone: (415) 488-9883

RECAP
c/o R. Wayne Griffiths
3205 Northwood Drive, Suite 209
Concord, CA 94520
Phone: (510) 827-4077

UNCIRC
PO Box 52138
Pacific Grove, CA 93950
Phone: (408) 375-4326
Send SASE for information.

Notes

1. Bigelow, Jim, Ph. D., *The Joy of Uncircumcising,* Aptos, CA, Hourglass Book Publishing, 1992, p. 49.
2. *Ibid.*, pp. 41-44.
3. Patel, Hawa, "The Problem of Routine Circumcision," *Journal of the Canadian Medical Association*, vol. 95, no. 11, Sept. 10, 1966, pp. 577-578.

Chapter Eighteen

GOING ALL THE WAY

Some people consider that the ultimate in disguise is total suppression of the past and taking on a new identity. This practice is rooted in American tradition. During the era when there were hardly any doctors, hospitals, or birth certificates, it was easy for a person to claim almost any name he wished. Few written records of any sort existed, one reason being that few knew how to read or write. The high illiteracy rate alone made a bureaucracy like today's impossible.

People did not need licenses or liability insurance to ride horses. Few attended school, and few school records existed. Without photography or fingerprinting, establishing positive identification was almost impossible. Anyone stopped by a law officer might find that, even if he had a birth or baptismal certificate to show, the officer was unable to read it.

In such circumstances, it was easy for almost anyone to "pull up stakes" and move on to establish himself with a new name elsewhere. Some people did it for adventure, while others did it to flee a dark or unpleasant past. Contrary to legend, most people who flee do so for mundane reasons. Most are not running from murder charges, but from nagging wives, child support, or other debts.

With the increasing power of governments, and with technology providing police with enhanced ability to practice surveillance of the population, getting a fresh start has become much more difficult than previously. From birth, a person starts to leave a paperwork trail. There are hospital and health records, school records, employment and credit records, military service records, and sometimes even police records.

One of the effects of this papering of our lives is that today a person finds himself accepted more on the basis of his documentation than his personality. Paperwork is everything. A motorist stopped by a police officer has only to present his driver's license and pass a radio check with the national crime computer to be allowed to go on his way. A credit applicant doesn't get close scrutiny by the lender. Instead, he fills in a form which goes to another person whom he never meets, and this person checks the information against computerized records and provides his evaluation solely on the basis of the paperwork. In that sense, paperwork has become more important than the individual.

Ironically, governments have taken steps to subvert their own systems of paperwork identification. Historically, espionage agencies have done this in order to send agents into enemy territory, forging the enemy government's documents, providing their agents with clothing and personal items manufactured in the enemy's country, so that the agents may pass as enemy nationals. This is called providing "cover." People living under totalitarian regimes, or under enemy occupation, have had occasion to do this, either to promote their escapes or to survive in various underground movements.

Technically, providing cover doesn't usually involve physical disguise, because the fugitive doesn't remain in his home locale, but moves to another area. He doesn't have to fear recognition by an acquaintance. Most of the effort involves procuring new identity documents and adopting a new lifestyle, all the time keeping a low profile to avoid attracting notice.

Today in this country there are several categories of people who want to escape their pasts. One is the person who "runs away from home," emotionally drained by his old lifestyle, a very unhappy job, a nagging spouse, or the need to support children, and who seeks a fresh start in another part of the country.

Another category is the protected federal witness. Since Joseph Valachi, the first member of organized crime to break the code of silence (so the legend goes), there had been by 1977 at least 2,000 people relocated and given new identities to protect them from retaliation from organized crime after their courtroom testimony.[1] This program has been mostly successful. As we've already seen there have been increasing numbers of people relocated during the several decades the program has existed.

This program is worth a close look, because it shows the techniques and hazards of establishing a new identity in the real world. The Federal Witness Protection Program was established under Title V of the Omnibus Organized Crime Control Act of 1970 and is run by the United States Marshal's Service.[2] The witnesses, usually former members of organized crime "families," are provided with new identities, given funds for relocation, usually provided with a team of U.S. Marshals as bodyguards during the transition, helped to find jobs, and given various supporting services after relocation.

Contrary to some legends, the U.S. Marshal's Service doesn't use wholesale plastic surgery or other extreme measures. The Service simply transports witnesses and their families to another part of the country, where it assigns them new identities and provides documents to support their new roles. By and large, this program has been successful, and very few participants have been tracked down and killed by the mob.

One who was killed spectacularly was Joseph Bombacino, who was living in Tempe, Arizona, under the name of Joseph Nardi after his relocation. One Monday morning in 1974, at about 20 minutes after eight, residents near his apartment heard a loud explosion. In one house, hundreds of yards away, the windows and arcadia door rattled, and the cat jumped backward about three feet at the sound of the detonation. Running outside, the residents saw a huge ball of smoke rising into the clear morning sky.

Bombacino's Lincoln Continental was burned-out wreckage. The gasoline tank had ruptured, and flames licked the devastated car. The Fire Chief estimated that the equivalent of 15 sticks of dynamite had blown up the car. Bombacino normally checked under the hood before getting into his car, as a precaution, but the explosive charge had been wired to the brake lights, so that there was no warning as Bombacino started his engine. He had backed out of his parking space, touched his brake pedal, and then he went into orbit. Pieces of the car were blown over the roof of his building into the next parking bay, and other fragments went as far as the nearby freeway.[3]

This explosive gangland execution, which the police never solved, was not as much a failure of the program as a personal failure of Bombacino's. He steadfastly neglected to keep a low profile. Having found work with a local utility company, he stole some supplies, was detected, and lost his job. He then brought suit to get his job back, but made the cardinal error of filing suit under his real name. This destroyed his carefully constructed cover, and once his enemies located him, setting up the "hit" was simple. The person who planted the bomb during the night was probably on the way out of town by the time it exploded.

Nuts and Bolts

Establishing a new identity in the United States is not hard. Most of the documentation isn't hard to obtain, even without help from a government agency. The procedure for obtaining a new birth certificate, known to secret agents, police, and criminals for years, first got wide prominence in Fredrick Forsyth's novel, *Day of the Jackal.*[4] The basic procedure is to find someone of the same sex and age, but who died in infancy or early childhood, and send for the birth certificate.[5]

Going to a library to scan microfilm copies of old newspapers for obituary notices is the simple first step. It's certainly more practical than searching through graveyards.

The inevitable question comes up: "Why someone who died in childhood?" Assuming the identity of someone still alive entails a risk. The person may be wanted for a crime, or for less dramatic reasons such as bad debts or child support. There's also a slight risk of meeting someone who knows the real person, and who could cause trouble over the discrepancy. Finally, someone who grows up to adulthood leaves a paper trail, such as photographs in school yearbooks.

Using a birth certificate as a base, it's easy to obtain other identity documents. For example, it's not even necessary to appear in person to obtain a Social Security card, if the applicant is under 18 years of age. Claiming to be under 18 is a very practical and logical step, as the Social Security card does not list the cardholder's age. In any event, most employers never ask to see the applicant's Social Security card, although they do ask for the number.

Making up a fictitious Social Security number is the quick and dirty way to do it, as the bureaucratic paperwork is so slow, and laden with mistakes, that the government won't catch up with the discrepancy for weeks or months, if ever. What helps is that many people make mistakes in listing their Social Security numbers. Giving a false Social Security number to an employer will not automatically bring federal agents to your door when the Social Security Administration discovers the discrepancy. They'll simply call or write your employer, and if you're still employed there he'll ask you if you gave him the correct number. If you sought only a temporary job, you may never be queried.

Obtaining a driver's license is almost as easy. A birth or baptismal certificate is usually all the proof of identity the authorities require, and a baptismal certificate is even easier to acquire than a birth certificate, as religious supply stores sell blanks.[6]

It's equally easy to obtain other government documents, such as a library card, resale and transaction tax license, etc., Easier still is the purchase of business cards, to help set up a false front for a new identity. These are very effective, considering their low cost and the ease of having them printed. Printers never check on business card customers, and it's easy to order business cards with the name of a non-existent company, or a false name and title attached to a real and well-known one.

Privately issued documents, such as credit cards, are another story. Companies issuing these are not satisfied with mere proof of identity, but want a credit history. This isn't as easy to falsify, because it's necessary to build it up from scratch. A way of doing this is detailed in one source.[7]

This brings us to one aspect of building up a new identity that's rarely discussed because it's a serious problem that doesn't lend itself to quick and easy solutions. This is "backstopping," putting into place the references and sources necessary to lend veracity to a new persona.

Backstopping documents requires leverage that the private individual usually lacks. It's relatively easy to forge a driver's license with a Polaroid camera, but if a police officer checks it out by radio with the motor vehicle bureau, he'll find out that there's no such license issued. It's necessary to backstop such documents to enable them to sustain a detailed investigation, such as a credit or security check, in which an investigator will contact the various sources normally listed in an application to verify the information.

Every real person has a history — where he went to school or church, previous employment, residences, etc. This is the most vulnerable point for a runaway, for only the real history exists, not the one relating to the new identity. Someone with a new identity can list a certain school on an employment application, but if an investigator contacts the school he'll learn that no such person attended. Even the most superficial background check will disclose the gaps.

The implications of this point are serious. A person taking on a new identity won't be able to obtain certain types of employment, and may be limited to menial jobs and those which don't demand a reference check. However, many employers, especially the small ones, don't have the time or inclination to check out all of the details and references demanded on employment applications. In any event, most take the viewpoint that what counts is performance on the job, and they usually hire a new employee with the reservation that if he doesn't work out, he's history. This is especially true of manual trades such as construction, printing, and other work which is well-paid and results in a tangible product. A new employee's skill is easy to assess quickly, and the employer can make an early determination regarding the new hire's job performance.

Employment with any level of government usually carries with it a background check. Other occupations, such as those in the medical field, also require background checks, although often not as formal or thorough. In fact, several hospital employees have turned out to be serial killers under suspicion at their previous jobs, but these suspicions didn't percolate through to their new employers.[8] However, a doctor, nurse, or lawyer cannot simply run away and continue to practice under another name. A license is involved, and the person applying for one must list his life story.

The Federal Witness Protection Program does backstop new identities to a certain extent. A cooperative college in the Midwest did, upon the request of the Justice Department, insert the appropriate papers into its records to support a witness's claim of having studied there. Various companies and individuals around the country will, upon request, serve as references for some of these witnesses. Yet these measures won't withstand a thorough background investigation, such as those used for security clearances.

A security clearance, despite what some people believe, doesn't apply only to government jobs, but is also necessary for civilians working for companies engaged in sensitive military contracts. This is stipulated by the Department of Defense, as part of the Defense Industrial Security Program. Employees seeking to work on classified projects must fill out clearance applications and submit to investigation, which is usually painless but very thorough. The application requires the employee to list all previous addresses, all schools attended, previous employments, criminal records, if any, and all family members. For some higher-level clearances, he must also submit his fingerprints.

An investigator will contact every school listed, in person, by phone, or by mail, to verify the record and obtain additional information. An investigator will also contact neighbors at each address listed, seeking information which might not show up on the application or other official records. An alcoholic, for example, might never have been arrested for drunk driving or disorderly conduct, yet his alcoholic fog might be obvious to his neighbors. The investigator will try to confirm many details, such as the names of the applicant's spouse or children, or the make of car driven. The investigator will also probe for other derogatory information, such as whether or not the applicant fights with his wife or neighbors. From this quick look at the process involved in granting security clearances, we can see that it doesn't require exotic techniques, such as polygraphs and drug-enhanced interviews, but simple and routine digging of the sort that even private individuals can do.

Some private employers, especially major corporations with large personnel and security departments, devote as much time and effort to employee verification as does the government. They follow the same procedures and obtain the same sort of information. While they lack the government's official status, their investigations can usually uncover the same sort of information. The common approach is to tell the interviewee frankly that they're conducting a pre-employment check, and this usually elicits cooperation.

It's important to emphasize that the major effort in background investigation doesn't involve polygraph tests, wiretapping, or other intrusive and possibly illegal methods. Most of the effort, as we've seen, goes into simple but time consuming checking of verifiable details. Such an investigation will defeat a new identity established without thorough backstopping, which we've seen is extraordinarily difficult to establish.

We can draw certain conclusions from this. It's easier to establish a new identity earlier in life, when there are fewer details open to investigation. Establishing a new identity requires not only documents, but time, and the more time available, the deeper the cover can be. It's very difficult for a 50-year-old man to start over again, especially if he has to leave his former life behind and create a new history for himself.

It can be done, and there have been some exceptional cases of brilliant impostors who passed themselves off as doctors and even performed surgery, until they were caught. This is rare, and these extraordinary instances are more a reflection of the stupidity and carelessness of medical school and hospital administrators than an indication of how easy it is. It is not easy, and getting away with an exceptionally bold impersonation requires luck as well as skill.

To "drop out" usually requires a change in lifestyle as well as a change in name. Much depends on the reason for eloping. Someone fleeing possible retaliation from organized crime has more reason to make a complete break than someone evading an unhappy marriage.

Often, a change of lifestyle includes a change of occupation. If the runaway is a professional person, he'll no longer be able to practice. Certain other occupations also carry paperwork trails the successful eloper must break. A machinist, plumber, carpenter, or painter may have a union card, without which he cannot work in many states. A union card is a link to the past. In many labor unions, obtaining a new card requires a considerable initiation fee, and proof of experience in the field. This is why relocating to a "right to work" state, in which lack of union membership is not a bar to employment, may be attractive. However, "right to work" states tend to have lower wages, and this may be an important consideration.

To break all connections with the past, it's necessary to study how an investigator tracing a fugitive would carry out his search. As a start, the investigator would interview relatives, friends, acquaintances, fellow employees, and neighbors to obtain details about his target's personal life. This would include hobbies, membership in clubs and other associations, reading habits, and other leisure activities. The investigator would try to trace him through his contacts with family and friends. Letters and telephone calls could serve as leads. An obvious example is a letter with the target's handwriting and return address on the envelope.

Breaking with the past is more difficult with increasing status and economic affluence. Someone with large stock holdings would want to collect dividends, and these would provide a direct paper trail to his door. Even those with modest roots tend to keep a part of their past with them, such as continuing to communicate with family members and close friends.

Preparing for the change ahead of time is an important step in avoiding a trace. The person planning to elope should sell all of his holdings, and take the cash or re-establish property and stock holdings under a new identity. He should also arrange to communicate through a system of mail drops.[9] The telephone is also useful as a means of hard-to-trace communication, but only if the fugitive avoids making long-distance calls from his home phone. A new wrinkle in telephone communication is "Caller I.D.," now used in several states.

Caller I.D. is a system which displays the caller's number on a screen while the phone is ringing. The telephone subscriber knows, therefore, the number from which the call is coming before picking up the phone. This makes it slightly more difficult for harassing telephone callers or others wanting to conceal their identities, as they have to use public phones to avoid being traced.

A basic rule for the fugitive is not to release his new name and address to anyone from his past. He should be aware that investigators have ruses with which they can pry information from someone whom the fugitive trusted.

He should also look at his hobbies and other activities. Membership in a sport association could give him away, especially if the association's publication goes to his new address. Any connection with an organization with a membership list small enough to make checking on new members practical can betray him if he resumes his membership under his new name. So can an unusual hobby.

Much depends on how important the fugitive is to the party trying to find him. With enough time and effort, there's a reasonable chance of a successful trace. In most cases, it's not practical to spend much time, effort, or money in unusually expensive ways of tracing a fugitive. While it's possible, for example, to have an investigator attend every chess match in the country in the hope of finding a fugitive known to be a chess fanatic, it's also prohibitively expensive.

Keeping a low profile is the other part of the technique. Knowing that his new I. D. will stand only limited scrutiny, the person will make an effort to avoid attracting attention. This includes the obvious, such as not running for public office or getting arrested, as well as subtleties such as avoiding situations in which he might have his photograph published in a newspaper. This can happen at a public function or if he associates with prominent and newsworthy people. In small towns, this can also happen if he joins a club. Various "service" and "social" clubs often invite a photographer from the local newspaper to take pictures of awards ceremonies and other events which they consider newsworthy. Clubs follow a pattern of bestowing awards, not necessarily on their own members, for various real or imagined services and contributions to the club or community. In this, they're so prolific that often the only way to avoid receiving an award is to commit suicide.

"Man in the Street" newspaper or TV interviews are another hazard. Any sort of activity leading to unwanted publicity can betray a cover. This is why it's important to be well-informed about local surroundings and customs. For example, a fugitive who joins a company that holds an employee picnic every year, or gives awards for long service, may also have media coverage. This is especially true in small or "company" towns. In one sense, the danger is limited, for such "news" doesn't go out on the wire service or network TV. Dissemination is local, apart from a few out-of-town mail subscriptions.

Local baseball teams and bowling tournaments often get coverage in local media. Sports news tends to get wider dissemination than club or company affairs. Attending local sporting events isn't necessarily hazardous, but it's important to be aware that photographers often get part of the crowd in the background while covering plays. One face in the crowd, among many, isn't easy to recognize, especially when diffused by a half-tone screen or TV raster. If small enough, it becomes indistinguishable from many others.

Being a participant definitely brings greater chances of unwanted publicity. One man, a contestant in a pistol match, was aware that the local TV station was covering the event, but because the TV cameraman was using a zoom lens, remained unaware that he was one of the stars of the show until he saw himself on the 10 o'clock news.

Paying attention to all of the details of relocation and a new identity requires not only ability, but emotional stamina. Not everyone can do it. To those who have never led an underground existence, it may seem adventurous, even romantic. It isn't. It's often dreary, and there are moments when the fugitive wonders if the future is really better than what he left behind.

Notes

1. Fred Graham, *The Alias Program*, Boston, Little, Brown, & Company, 1977. This is a fairly thorough book, written mainly in narrative style, dealing with the efforts of the U.S. Department of Justice to relocate witnesses under new identities. To the careful reader, the book shows how assuming a new identity requires a change in lifestyle as well as supporting documents. While writers of crime and espionage novels often mention plastic surgery to give the person

a new appearance and new fingerprints, the truth is simpler and far less dramatic.

2. *Ibid.*, p. 47.

3. Witnessed by the author, who lived nearby at the time.

4. Frederick Forsyth, *The Day of the Jackal,* NY, The Viking Press, 1971.

5. *The Paper Trip*, Fountain Valley, CA, Eden Press, 1971, and *New I. D. in America*, Boulder, CO, Paladin Press, 1983. Both books provide valuable hands-on information regarding how to procure new I. D. *The Paper Trip* has a second volume, with lists of government offices from which to obtain various identity documents, and a section on graphics, with reproductions of official seals to aid in outright forgery.

    New I. D. in America has a lot of practical information on the mechanics of establishing a new identity, and the book is short and sweet. While there's little reference information, such as the list of birth registrars found in *The Paper Trip II,* the book tells the reader how to find such information. More importantly, it tells how to break a trail, and there is even a chapter on how an investigator might try to trace a wanted person.

6. *New I. D. in America*, pp. 9-29.

7. *Ibid.,* p. 81.

8. Newton, Michael, *Hunting Humans, An Encyclopedia of Modern Serial Killers*, Port Townsend, WA, Loompanics Unlimited, 1990, pp. 177-178. The case of Genene Jones is typical and instructive. Jones was a suspect in the mysterious deaths of 47 children in Bexar County Hospital in Texas, but she left to go to work for a pediatrician in nearby Kerrville, Texas. In Kerrville, she was involved in more deaths, the pediatrician having hired Jones despite being "indirectly cautioned" by hospital administrators. In fact, this isn't surprising, because a massive lawsuit awaits a

former employer who accuses an employee of a felony without proof.
9. *New I. D. in America,* p. 49.

Chapter Nineteen

FUTURISTIC PROSPECTS

In our industrialized society, there are certain legitimate needs for technological methods of personal identification. We have a system of recording births, for example, to establish citizenship. Credit cards of various types are a help in making purchases. However, this isn't the whole story. Both government and private organizations use modern methods of identification to establish control over individuals. The police and tax collection and enforcement agencies are good examples.

In many countries, the government requires everyone over a certain age to carry a national identity card. This is mainly true in totalitarian countries, but it's happened in more liberal regimes during wartime. In some countries, citizens must register every change of address with the police. Again, this isn't an exclusively totalitarian practice, as we find it in countries such as France, Italy and Switzerland.

The United States is one of the few countries which has never had a Single Universal Identifier, or SUI — a personal identity document required as part of the personal paperwork that every person must carry with him. As Americans, we don't have to carry a driver's license if we're not driving, we don't have to show a credit card if we pay cash, and even draft cards are usually temporary, existing mainly during wartime or national emergency.

The reason is that we have a tradition of personal freedom that most of us consider very important. From this country's earliest days, Americans feared and distrusted a powerful central government, and resisted any measures which seemed designed to impose totalitarianism or bureaucratic control over their whereabouts or conduct. However, government control and other intrusions have been slipping in through the back door.

Today, the picture is somewhat different, and identification paperwork has crept up on us, not so much through the government, but by private organizations. We have to disclose personal information when applying for employment or credit, and this information goes into a computer, to be scrutinized by faceless people we never meet. We have little or no control over what the organizations do with the information we provide, and it often returns to haunt us later. We resent it, but there's little we can do. The same "freedom" which enables us to refuse to divulge personal information allows an employer or credit organization to refuse us employment or credit as the penalty for non-cooperation.

The government concerns us most, because in the end the government has more coercive power than any private organization. A loan company can't execute those who default on payments, but there are many examples of such extraordinary exercise of power by some of the world's governments.

Some government functionaries favor more control over the individual, and technology is on their side. Many police officials, for example, have privately expressed the opinion that all babies should be fingerprinted at birth, with the prints kept on file by a national police organization or in a data bank accessible to police agencies. The reason this has not yet come about is the concern of both citizens and legislators with the "Big Brother" implications of such a plan. The current controversy over fingerprinting small children as an aid to identification in case of kidnapping, disaster, or other mishaps, is an example of how Americans feel about what they see as an infringement of their freedom.

With new technologies will come more ways of keeping track of individuals, and this poses severe social and Constitutional problems.[1] No doubt, there will be strong objections to any plan for national identification, and some of the new ideas will only come about in limited ways, in carefully selected cases.

One such technological innovation is a form of electronic house arrest, using a bracelet that emits a radio signal picked up by a nearby receiver. This serves as an innovative type of parole or probation, in which the receiver is linked to the local probation office. If the probationer travels more than a certain distance from the receiver the signal fades, and the probation officer knows that the probationer has violated the terms of parole or probation by leaving the area. A receiver in the parolee's home allows enforcement of a curfew. Another use is control over the hours the person is absent, allowing him to go to work, but alerting the probation office if he's not back at a specified time.

This has been easy to introduce because in a certain sense, a lawbreaker forfeits both his rights and public sympathy once convicted and sentenced. As a practical matter, serving a sentence at home is less onerous than serving hard time behind bars. For the most part, the convicts don't object. There are, however, more devices on the horizon — devices not even imagined by science fiction writers years ago.

It's not hard to imagine a device locked onto the wrist of every citizen, containing a transmitter sending out coded pulses identifying the wearer. More simply, a magnetic strip on a bracelet could serve as a unique identifier, without the expense of a transmitter. Such devices would defeat any disguise.

There are more sinister and objectionable methods available. Newborns might not only be fingerprinted, but have tiny transmitters surgically implanted. These would remain with each newborn throughout life, not only for identification, but to pinpoint his location through a network of receivers. An implanted device would be more tamper-proof and harder to remove than a bracelet.

The important point is that these devices are not science fiction. Today's technology allows building them. Implanted electronics have existed for years in pacemakers. A grid network of radio transceivers exists today to support cellular phones.

The only obstacles to implementing personal implanted radio transmitters are their questionable legality and strong lack of public acceptance. Low-tech methods of permanent identification, such as tattoos, have existed for years.[2] Tattoos have never been applied universally in this country, but have seen use in other parts of the world, their most notorious application being to identify concentration camp inmates.

Each device brings its countermeasures, and there's no reason to think that futuristic devices might not be vulnerable. Let's look at a few scenarios to get an impression of the possibilities:

- A prison administration uses bracelets emitting radio signals to keep track of "trustees" allowed to work outside the prison walls. A fence surrounds the area in which they're confined, but this isn't a high barbed-wire fence. It's a low one with antennas every few yards. Anyone approaching the fence while wearing a bracelet would activate an alarm, summoning guards. One prisoner, planning an escape, removes his bracelet with a saw or bolt-cutter, and vaults undetected over the fence.

- With the government requiring citizens to wear magnetic rings, counterfeiting operations begin. Electronic forgers using sophisticated equipment record false information onto rings for a fee. This allows people to assume false identities even more easily than during the old days of conventional disguises. As authorities consider bracelets infallible, they have the person to be identified place his wrist near a magnetic reader, and accept the reading without scrutinizing the person further. Electronic engineers reprogram their bracelets with absurd names, while retaining correct identification numbers, and pass through security checks into restricted work areas. They keep this joke up for several weeks before being detected.

- Everyone has a miniature transmitter implanted at birth. This allows the government to pinpoint everyone's position at all times, and to track each person's whereabouts throughout his life, preserving the records in a giant computer. While this aids police by identifying those near crime scenes, many people object to this Big Brotherism. A few bold experimenters find that they can deactivate their implants by exposing them to a short burst of microwaves — not enough to cook the tissue around the implant, but enough to fry the delicate microchips. The news gets around, and although the majority of citizens don't jam their implants, enough do to make the system partially unworkable.

• With each citizen carrying an implanted transmitter, a black market springs up to cater to those who want to tamper with their implants. Criminal gangs find it remarkably easy to circumvent the government's tracking system. Out of millions of receivers, located at hundred-yard intervals in a grid pattern all over the country, thousands are inoperable at a given moment because of defects, lightning strikes, power failures, and assorted other failures. Vandals also take their toll, and in some central city areas, receivers suffer sabotage as often as public telephones. The government employs large repair and maintenance crews to keep its electronic grid operating.

Criminals learn how easy it is to disable receivers near crime scenes. Small, portable microwave generators burn out the black boxes in seconds. Small hand-held jammers confuse the receivers. The simplest method is to hit the receiver with a hammer, smashing it beyond repair. The only disadvantage to using a hammer is that many receivers are mounted on poles or on the sides of buildings high enough to be hard to reach. The more aggressive criminals disable these with gunfire. The central computer cannot distinguish between a failure resulting from sabotage or other causes.

The technology exists. There are sophisticated means of establishing identity and location for each of us. There are also means to frustrate these techniques. Each measure inspires countermeasures. The balance shifts, first one way, then the other. How it will all turn out only the future will tell.

Notes

1. George H. Warfel, *Identification Technologies*, Springfield, IL, Charles C. Thomas, Publisher, 1979, pp. 20-31.
2. *Ibid.*, p. 182. The author seems to look forward eagerly to the prospect of implanted devices,

APPENDIX I:

CROSS-DRESSING AND SEX CHANGE

There have been a few instances of people disguising themselves as the opposite sex for other than erotic purposes. A sen-
sational case was that of Dr. Hawley Crippen, an American
living in England. In 1910, Dr. Crippen murdered his wife
Belle with poison, to free himself to give his attention to Ethel
Neve, a young lady who seemed more attractive. He buried his
wife's body in his basement, but unfortunately for him Scotland
Yard became interested in his wife's sudden disappearance and
one of their inspectors dug up the basement of Dr. Crippen's
house and discovered the remains.[1]

Meanwhile, Dr. Crippen and Ethel Neve had disappeared.
Ethel had bought a suit of boy's clothing and disguised herself
accordingly. Dr. Crippen, using the alias of "Robinson," had
booked passage for himself and his "son" on a passenger ship
bound across the Atlantic. By the time the voyage was under-
way, the ship's captain noticed something funny about the

Robinson "boy." The trousers were too tight in the rear, among other things. The news of Dr. Crippen's being wanted for investigation of murder was widespread and the captain sent a radio message to the British Police. The inspector on the case took a faster ship and intercepted Crippen and Ethel Neve before they were able to disembark in Quebec.

This was an unsuccessful attempt at cross-sex impersonation. There's hardly any way of knowing how successful other attempts have been, or even how many have occurred. We can make an educated guess and say that there must be few, for the simple reason that disguising oneself as a member of the same sex is much easier than trying to resemble the opposite sex.

Nevertheless, this course interests some people, and it's worth a quick look. Most large cities have one or more transvestite, or "TV" bars, not necessarily "gay" bars, in which those who like to make up as the opposite sex gather. In fact, transvestitism is a subculture in this country, although a small one.

The techniques of disguising a man as a woman are similar to make-up techniques used by women themselves. A man might want to tweeze his eyebrows if he's "beetle-browed," and foundation and face powder help soften the complexion. Shaving is a must. Lipstick is optional, although many women use it, more or less discreetly. Many also wear wigs.

Clothing isn't usually a problem, although there are specialty companies advertising in transsexual publications so that a "TV" who wants to order by mail may do so.[2] The entire range is available via mail order: dresses, blouses, sweaters, skirts and pants, jeans, suits, jackets, bags, cosmetics, furs, and even beard covers.

There are several publications catering to transvestites. Some are available over-the-counter in adult bookstores and sex shops. Others are by subscription only, perhaps because of inadequate over-the-counter demand. A list of publications is at the end of this appendix.[3]

The results of cross-dressing, judging by the illustrations appearing in "TV" publications, are not very good. Although some manage to create a good simulation of a woman in a photograph, most do not. It's one thing to look at a photograph of a person never seen before, and another to meet the person face to face. Simulating a woman requires more than a wig, some clothing, and make-up. In person, the simulation must be three-dimensional, and this is much more difficult to carry out, although some have done it extraordinarily well.

"Sex change" surgery is even more exotic. According to one prominent plastic surgeon in the field, "several thousand" such operations have taken place in this country. He considers this to be mainly self-image surgery, as those who apply for it state they feel they are trapped in the wrong gender. The cost is substantial and runs from $5,000 to more than $20,000, depending on the extent of the surgery, and includes hospitalization and incidentals. This is not usually covered by medical insurance, as insurance companies feel that this is cosmetic surgery, and therefore unnecessary.

How good are the cosmetic results? They vary. One plastic surgeon related a case of a man who had had a sex change operation, and in the doctor's words the job was "slick." This person used to present himself at a clinic in San Antonio regularly, with both real and imagined ailments, as he got a thrill from being examined by doctors and medical students. His counterfeit sex often went undetected.

As a practical matter, anyone who asked a plastic surgeon for sex reassignment surgery for disguise purposes would probably get a refusal. This refusal would be, in every sense, a reflection of cultural values rather than the result of considered medical judgment. Most surgeons would consider the reason given, disguise, as frivolous or irrational, although many such surgeons will accept the patient's feeling that he or she is 'trapped" in the wrong body. The surgery's the same; only the "reasons" differ, and this is hard to justify.

Again, as a purely practical matter, anyone considering sex reassignment surgery must count on a period of psychiatric evaluation that can easily last for two years. This will include psychological testing, and interviews with a psychiatrist. Much of this comes under the heading of "counseling."

The prelude to surgery is hormone injections to develop secondary sexual characteristics such as body hair distribution, and fat deposits in the appropriate places. This can affect the figure, although bone structure remains unchanged. While a man will retain his relatively broad shoulders and narrow hips, female hormones will bring about a deposit of fat on the hips, somewhat changing the body's contours.

Surgical techniques vary both in style and number. One common technique is to invert the skin of the penis and to implant it into the abdomen to simulate the vaginal barrel. The scrotal tissue is useful for constructing the external labia, as scrotal hair will simulate the pubic hairs on the labia majora.

A bizarre case of sexual reassignment surgery resulted after a boy whose penis was accidentally amputated during circumcision underwent sex reassignment surgery at the age of 18 months.[4] Raising him as a girl after the disastrous mutilation seemed the best choice for his parents, although the boy/girl will never be able to bear children.

For the most part, "sex change" surgery isn't practical as a means of disguise. Not only are the techniques crude, but there are easier ways to disguise oneself.

Notes

1. Bond, Raymond, Editor, *Handbook For Poisoners*, NY, Collier Books, 1951, pp. 37-40.
2. Sources of apparel and other items for cross-dressing are:

E.H.B. (Also operates under the name of "Especially For Me")
PO Box 1489
Ontario, CA 91862
Phone: (714) 946-6251
Fax: (714) 946-5500
    E.H.B. carries breast items, rubber pants, slips and other underwear, gloves, wigs, breast forms, and other TV items. Also publishes a catalog.

Laura Lee
PO Box 711
Farmingdale, NJ 07727-0711
Laura Lee advertises in various tabloids.

Versatile Fashions
PO Box 1051
Tustin, CA 92681
Phone: (714) 538-6498

Versatile Fashion's boutique is located at:
1925 E. Lincoln Avenue
Anaheim, CA 92805
Phone: (714) 776-1510

3. Publications and other media materials relating to transvestitism are available from:

Classic Publications
PO Box 2113
Apple Valley, CA 92307
    Classic sells erotic stories covering bondage and restraint.

Ground Zero Enterprises, Ltd.
PO Box 7575
LaVerne, CA 91750
   Publishes *TV Sexcapades,* a tabloid for transvestites that includes personal ads, phone hot lines, and sources of materials and supplies.

Letro Limited
PO Box 2966
Mission Viejo, CA 92690
   Letro Limited sells "adult" videos, covering the following topics: Hermaphrodites, She-Male, TV, Pregnant, Amateur, B&D, and other hard to find videos.

Tania Volen
PO Box 280
Tennent, NJ 07763-0280
   Tania Volen publishes *Dateline, Discipline, Femanine, Leather and Lace, Players, The Sophisticate, TransForm,* and *The Transvestian.*
4. John Money, Ph. D., and Patricia Tucker, *Sexual Signatures*, Boston, Little, Brown & Co. 1975, p. 91.

APPENDIX II:

FALSIFYING FINGERPRINTS

There are several methods of erasing or falsifying fingerprints. Let's examine each closely and draw conclusions regarding their practicality.

As any plastic surgeon will attest, "dermabrasion," or sandpapering skin, will remove marks, irregularities, and even fingerprints. Some criminals found it possible to sandpaper their finger pads and remove the ridges that form their fingerprints. Removing the top layers of skin leaves a smooth surface that won't deposit a fingerprint pattern. However, these ridges grow back within a few weeks, the exact time depending on how much skin was abraded. (See Figure A-1.)

Another technique is to sand the skin until the full thickness is removed, or to remove the full thickness surgically. Removing the underlying skin layers ensures that the ridges never grow back. The area either fills in with scar tissue, or if the removal is surgical, the surgeon can apply graft from another area of the body.

There's a catch, though. Both of these full-thickness removal methods leave the person with scars that will be far more distinctive than the original fingerprints. In the case of a criminal suspect, police will investigate very thoroughly anyone who shows evidence of surgical tampering with fingerprints. In that sense, it's counterproductive because it attracts as much attention as a clown suit at a funeral. If the purpose is to avoid leaving fingerprints at a crime scene, it's much easier to wear gloves than to undertake abrasive or surgical fingerprint modification.

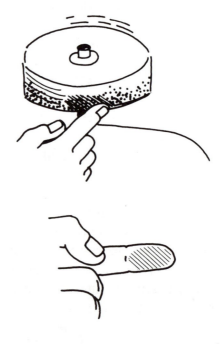

Figure A-1

Removing fingerprints with a drum sander. This method leaves smooth fingertips, although the prints grow back within a few weeks.

If you wear gloves to avoid leaving fingerprints, make sure to take them away with you! Today, it's possible to develop fingerprints from the insides of gloves, especially plastic or rubber gloves. If you leave the gloves anywhere they might be found, you risk leaving your prints behind.

Yet another way to avoid leaving fingerprints is to coat the fingertips with paint or household cement. This fills in the grooves between the ridges and masks the characteristic pattern. Unfortunately, such a coating makes the skin smoother, and this can be a disadvantage because fingerprint ridges help to grip objects.

There is a method of falsifying fingerprints which works well under controlled conditions, but its use in the field sometimes poses problems. It's possible to make casts of the finger-pad ridges with liquid latex, obtainable from a make-up supply house. (See Figure A-2.) The technique works as follows:

1. With a brush, apply a thin layer of latex to the pad of the finger, carefully coating the whole surface from the wrinkle of the finger-joint to just below the nail. Allow to dry for at least two minutes. The latex, milky when applied, turns clear when dry.

2. Apply another layer and allow to dry.

3. Apply another coat, let dry, and brush on a fourth coat. To obtain a casting that you can peel off without tearing, at least four coats are necessary. For best results, four thin coats are better than two or three thick ones. The most important coat, though, is the first, which must be as thin as possible and worked in well with the brush to fill the spaces between the ridges.

4. Once the latex casting is thoroughly dry, peel it off with tweezers, starting at one corner. If you've applied the latex well and allowed it to dry long enough, it should peel off without tearing.

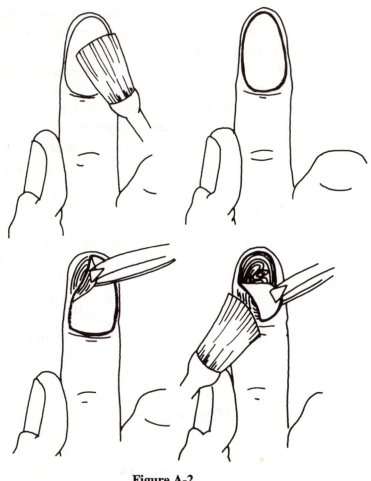

Figure A-2

*False fingerprints can be created by using liquid latex,
then gluing them to the fingertips.*

5. Two possible problems are wrinkling and tearing. If the la-
    tex is too thin because you applied too few layers, it will
    tend to fold over on itself and wrinkle. Tearing, on the other
    hand, happens when the latex sticks to the skin. This tends
    to happen with dry skin, and one cure is to use a "release

agent," an oily substance that reduces adhesion. The best to use is the natural oils found on the skin. Rub your fingertip on your forehead or the side of your nose before you begin.

6. The result will be a flexible cast of your fingerprint, which you can cement to another finger with rubber cement, spirit gum, or any other adhesive you've found safe to use on your skin. Your fingerprint will be flopped left-to-right, but this doesn't matter because it will leave a clear print. Small imperfections also don't matter, because surfaces you touch are likely to have coatings of dust which impede leaving perfect prints, anyway. In any case, most people's fingertips have small abrasions and imperfections.

7. Depositing fingerprints on an object requires a light film of sweat and skin oil on the casting. Skin normally secretes these, but the latex casting won't. This is why it's necessary to rub the finger with the false print on your nose or forehead.

   One problem with this method is obtaining suitable casts from unwilling subjects. If your purpose is to leave someone else's prints, trying to cast his prints without his knowledge or permission is impractical. Drugs and hypnosis work only in spy novels.

   As a practical matter, if you want to leave a person's fingerprints at a crime scene, the easy way to do it is to leave an object, such as a glass or handgun, that he's handled. Once you've obtained such an object, pack it carefully in cotton to transport it to the scene.

8. Another problem is that this method will never pass when having your fingerprints taken, because the fingerprint technician is bound to notice the castings cemented to your fingertips. It's next to impossible to cement them perfectly. There may be a rolled or raised edge, and it may not be possible to match the skin color perfectly. Another problem is that the ink used for fingerprinting is sticky, and unless

the castings are solidly attached, they may come off, remaining on the glass plate on which the technician spreads the ink.

Falsifying fingerprints is possible, from a strictly technical point of view. Making practical use of them is often unworkable, and it's easier to use other methods.

Appendix III:

IMPERSONATION

Impersonating a specific individual is probably the most difficult part of disguise. We'll look at a few specifics and see why.

Let's begin with a hypothetical example. If a man appeared and stated that he was George Washington, we'd laugh at him even if he looked the part perfectly to the last detail, such as wig, clothing, etc. However, the interesting fact is that, no matter how absurd his claim was, we could not prove that this impostor was not George Washington. The reasons for this teach us a lot about the nitty-gritty of impersonation:

1. There are no photographs of George Washington. There are some portraits and busts, but most don't resemble each other. We still don't know for sure exactly how George Washington looked.

2. Even the few physical details we know about George Washington could fit many men. We know, for example,

that he was a large man, well over six feet in height, but we don't know exactly how tall he was or how much he weighed. The rulers in use then were not standardized, as there was no nationally recognized standard for measurement, and consequently we can't rely upon recorded data.

3. No fingerprints of George Washington are on file, as fingerprinting was not in use then.

4. Nobody who knew George Washington is alive today. Therefore, nobody could verify or deny that our hypothetical Washington looked the part, had the same voice, the same gait, and had the same behavioral characteristics as the original. Without television, motion pictures, or sound recording, we really know very little about George Washington.

5. None of the other techniques sometimes used to tell one person from another existed then. We don't have George Washington's X-rays on file, nor do we know his blood type. Even the details of medical treatment he received during his life are sketchy.

From this we can see that although we simply would not believe a person who claimed to be someone who has been dead for two centuries, we could not disprove his claim. It's clear that a person's identity is composed of characteristics in several dimensions, and that a face or an I. D. card isn't enough.

Anyone seeking to impersonate another must consider two factors:

1. The closeness of the match attainable.

2. The closeness of the scrutiny.

Many people impersonate others every day, an example being an actor who plays a historical figure in a play or movie. A check forger using a forged or stolen driver's license to pass himself off as someone else is also an impersonator. The actor is a medium-grade impersonator, because he takes the time and trouble to make up as his character, and studies and mimics his mannerisms. The forger is a low-grade impersonator because he tries only to pass himself off to a stranger who doesn't know the original person.

The foremost fact about an actor playing a part is that he does so under closely controlled conditions. He doesn't have to pass truly critical examination and, realistically, he doesn't try to convince people that he is really the person he's playing. Audiences suspend their disbelief, which makes it relatively easy to play a role on stage or screen compared to real life under close scrutiny. Richard Corson's book on stage make-up shows Hal Holbrook making up as Mark Twain, and Peter Falk disguising himself as Stalin.[1] The accompanying text brings out the fact that make-up takes hours to apply, and the photographs depict the elaborate steps required.

Both Holbrook and Falk are professional actors, and we cannot fault their skills. However, if Peter Falk were to walk into the Kremlin and claim that he was Stalin, he'd have a great deal of trouble convincing anyone of his authenticity.

Audiences often suspend their disbelief to the extent that they don't expect an actor to be an exact match. Both Robert Duvall and Andrew Duggan have played Dwight D. Eisenhower, although they're physically disparate. Duvall is of average height at most, Eisenhower was about 5' 10", while Duggan is well over six feet. Both have facial bone structures somewhat like Eisenhower's, but neither is an exact match. Nevertheless, both performed successfully.

The reason that performances are successful is, as we've seen, that conditions are carefully controlled. In a film or TV production, lighting and camera angles are under control to show the actors best. On stage, audiences don't get close enough to examine the actors carefully.

Sometimes the discrepancies can be glaring, yet audiences still accept the performances. George C. Scott's rendition of Patton, for example, conflicted with the real Patton in several important ways. Scott's booming voice was very unlike the real Patton's high-pitched one. Yet, the performance carried the audience and won George C. Scott an Academy Award.

The film *Bonnie and Clyde* was a misrepresentation of reality in several ways, including how the characters looked. Faye Dunaway and Warren Beatty produced glitzy and glamorous renditions of the dowdy Bonnie and the drab, sullen Clyde, but the film was still a success.

Hal Holbrook had an easier time imitating Mark Twain. Much of Twain's face was covered with whiskers, and there's nobody alive who remembers the real Twain.

Anyone who has known identical twins knows that it's often difficult to tell them apart. Some twins dress alike and impersonate each other as a joke on family members and friends. This is a classic example of closeness of match, in which little or no effort is necessary to pass oneself off as the other. Yet, no set of identical twins has yet had identical fingerprints, which shows that limitations exist.

One popular saying is that each of us has a double somewhere in the world. Some people have found this to be true, because occasionally look-alikes have encountered each other.

It was just such a set of look-alikes that led to the Bertillon System's downfall. The Bertillon System was a set of measurements of several body dimensions and facial photographs, used to identify criminals during the late 19th century and the early part of the 20th. In 1903, a man named Will West arrived at Leavenworth Penitentiary to begin his term. The technician who classified him according to the Bertillon System knew that he'd seen West before. It turned out that there was another West in Leavenworth, and his given name was William. To carry the coincidence further, his measurements, facial features, and general appearance were so similar to the other West that they seemed to be doubles, although their fingerprints were different.

Despite the close similarity, they weren't related, and didn't even know each other.[2]

Some security services have used doubles either to play a game of deception against an enemy, or as a security measure for protection of a leader. The widely-publicized case of Field Marshal Montgomery's double is one example. A small-time actor was employed to impersonate Montgomery and mislead the Germans as to his whereabouts. There have also been un-verified reports of a Hitler double used to impede assassination attempts, and supposedly Winston Churchill had a double for the same purpose.

Using a double for protective purposes is common, al-though these are not high-grade impersonations. A Presidential motorcade that has several similar limousines, with similarly dressed men riding inside, is one common example. A close look would quickly uncover the impostors, but a potential as-sassin scrutinizing the motorcade from afar would be uncertain.

Spy novels are full of instances of enemy agents impersonating government officials. In 1915, *The Thirty-Nine Steps*, by John Buchan, appeared. In this story, a German master spy who was also a master of disguise penetrated a meeting of government officials by impersonating "Lord Alloa," one of the participants. He got in and out undetected, despite the fact that his eyes were very distinctive and he had a finger missing. The other participants, who had known Lord Alloa for years, some-how overlooked these discrepancies.[3]

Fictional impersonators in the employ of foreign powers are all masters of disguise, according to their creators. Sometimes they're aided by plastic surgery, as in a rash of cold-war novels. This is pure fiction.

In real life, there have been several Soviet agents who have impersonated citizens of the Western Powers, but not in the way spy novels depict. Konon Molody, the Soviet agent who passed as "Gordon Lonsdale" in a famous British spy case three decades ago, took the identity of a person who had been born in Canada but had been taken back to Eastern Europe before the start of World War II. The real Gordon Lonsdale vanished in the storm of the war. Molody simply claimed to be Gordon Lonsdale, and didn't have a difficult time of it, because nobody on this side of the Iron Curtain had known the real Lonsdale as an adult. Molody/Lonsdale didn't apply for a government job that would have brought him under close scrutiny, but immigrated to England under his alias and served as a go-between, contacting agents in the British Government who passed him information for the Soviet Intelligence Service. "Lonsdale" never had any difficulties with his impersonation as such, but the British Security Service traced him through his spying. British police agents followed one of the traitors who was passing him information and arrested them both as they were handing over the material.

Molody's impersonation did not fall apart until after his arrest, and then only by a curious development. British police subjected him to very close inspection, including an examination by a doctor. Comparing medical records, they found that the real Lonsdale had been circumcised as a boy in Canada, but the "Lonsdale" they had in the cell was intact.

The closeness of the scrutiny is the most important factor determining the difficulties and the chances of success of the impersonation. In many cases, the impostor doesn't have to fool anyone who knows the subject well, and doesn't have to pass any rigorous security checks.

Thirty years ago, in Fairfield, CT, an employee in a closely-guarded defense plant substituted a photo of Adolf Hitler for his own on his identification badge. Daily, he passed by gate guards while entering and leaving the plant. During the workday, he mingled with fellow employees and did his work in a normal manner. After one week, someone noticed something wrong, and his little joke came to an end.

This is a good example of how "security measures" often don't provide much real security. A photo I.D. badge should be a safeguard against anyone who doesn't resemble the photo, but when bored and careless security guards examine thousands of badges daily, their effectiveness drops.

A photo I.D. badge is just the beginning of the task in overcoming security measures, and making an impersonation succeed. While it may be easy to carry out an impersonation against someone who doesn't know the subject well or has never met him, it's another matter to pass inspection by friend and family. Not only must physical features match, but the impersonator must correspond in other ways:

Voice quality and speech pattern.

Expression — Some people characteristically look happy or sad.

Clothing usually worn by the subject. Some people's clothing is a trademark.

Walk and other features of gait and posture.

Content of conversation — Someone who knows nothing about baseball would have a hard time if the subject were an avid baseball fan.

Mental state — Some people have sunny dispositions, while others are characteristically gloomy. The impersonator must mimic this too.

Political or social opinion — If an impersonator, mimicking a certain subject with conservative opinions, begins speaking like a liberal, friends and acquaintances will notice this immediately. This is true even when mimicking a subject to people who have never met him. It would be out of place, for example, for someone disguised as a Roman Catholic priest to speak out in favor of abortion.

Sexual behavior — This is essential if the subject is married or has a regular sexual relationship with another person. This is one reason why Soviet agents have usually assumed the identities of people who were unattached, in one case a Roman Catholic priest.

From this very incomplete list, we can see how difficult it can be to manage an impersonation. There are too many dimensions to a human being to copy all of them beyond detection. An impersonator must study his subject well, and mimic not only his appearance but his behavior to fool even casual acquaintances. Passing through a security check, background investigation, or gaining access to a restricted area can be even harder.

To understand the obstacles, let's look at another hypothetical case, that of a company which does secret government work, has an intelligent security director, and well-paid, well-trained, and well-motivated guards manning an effective access control system.

We must recognize at the outset that the hypothetical organization described here probably doesn't have a real life counterpart anywhere in the world, and certainly not in the Western world. In real life, people with repetitive jobs that require vigilance and intelligence become bored, or even burned out after a while, and their alertness falls. It's also true that security measures are not part of the production process, add nothing to the companies' profits, and fall into the category called "overhead." Business executives, even those doing business with the Pentagon, tend to cut corners on security, doing only the bare minimum regulations require, and spending as little as possible on personnel and equipment. In real life, the main requirement for a security officer is willingness to work for low pay. In some instances, the company "security officer" is a person who works in another department, carrying out security duties part-time in addition to other work. This is especially true in small companies.

Our hypothetical agent applies for a job at our hypothetical company. As a start, he has to fill out the usual employment application and a security questionnaire. The questionnaire asks for his life history, including his grandmother's maiden name. Before he gets his security clearance, which allows him to enter restricted areas, his paperwork will be investigated by several Defense Industrial Security Clearance Office (DISCO) investigators to verify the details. The investigators' reports go to an evaluator, who reads them and then either passes or rejects the applicant.

As part of the initial procedure, the applicant must furnish his fingerprints. He may do this at the local police department, or the security officer may take his fingerprints on company premises. This is to ensure that the fingerprints are actually the applicant's, and not a substitution. A government investigator will check out the prints against others on file. If the applicant has been in the armed forces, or the police, his fingerprints will be on file with the appropriate agency. If he's been convicted of a felony, his prints will be in FBI files. The fingerprint check is both to prove that the applicant is who he says he is, and to discover a hidden past. Assuming that the records are in order, and that none are lost or misfiled, the check will be thorough.

During initial pre-employment processing the applicant will have a medical examination, which can be very thorough. In our hypothetical case, information recorded during the medical examination will be compared with the applicant's earlier medical records. If there are any discrepancies, such as blood type, this will provoke a closer investigation. If medical records show that the applicant had an appendectomy at age 15, but there's no corresponding scar on the applicant's abdomen, this is cause for concern.

As part of the final processing after clearance, the new employee will have to furnish several samples of his signature, pose for mug shots, and speak several specific words into a microphone, to provide identification data for the access control system. The security officer will issue him a tamper-resistant photo I.D. card, and a personal identification number to memorize.

Let's now consider the problems which an agent trying to impersonate an employee cleared to work in the high-security area has to face. First, he must be a close physical match, close enough to adjust his dimensions by shoe lifts or by diet, and his facial features should be close enough so that he can pass with minimal make-up. He'll also have to mimic the subject's walk and speech closely.

To gain access, he'll first have to obtain a security photo I.D. badge, by taking it from the subject or by forgery. If he succeeds, he'll be able to get by the gate guard. Upon entering the building, he'll have to sign in at the front desk, manned by a security guard who'll compare the signature with one on file.

Badges are color-coded, each color signifying clearance for a certain restricted area. Color codes also change periodically as an additional security measure, to prevent anyone finding a lost badge from using it for more than a limited time, and the impostor must have the right color. Color changes also make forgery that much more complicated.

At the high-security area, the impostor must go through several stages. First, he must sign in once more, this time on an electronic pad which records the rhythm of his signature. This is a device that's very hard to fool, as a forger may be able to reproduce his subject's signature personally, but will find it hard to do it with the same speed and rhythm.[4] This screens out forgers who have not watched the subject sign his name, or practiced the same speed and rhythm. In any case, it's doubtful that a forger would be able to duplicate the subject's speed and rhythm closely.

If our agent passes the test, he'll enter a compartment leading to the high-security area. This has a double set of doors, like an air lock, electronically interfaced so that only one door can open at a time. To open the outside door, our agent must insert his photo I.D. card into a slot with an electronic reader. The card has a magnetic stripe identifying the subject, and the information read goes to the central access control computer. However, the card does not open the door. To gain access, the agent must enter his Personal Identification Number (PIN) on a keypad. If he fails to key in the correct number, the door remains closed and a light goes on at the control panel on the guard's desk. If the agent keys in the correct number, the door opens to admit him, only to lock again once the agent is inside.

A significant detail is that the PIN is not magnetically recorded on the card, nor is any other security information. This prevents anyone, even if he has the equipment, from reading security information from the card. The card contains only the employee's name and company identification number, which enable the computer to recall and display the information on a monitor at the guard's console. The information about the employee's signature pattern remains in the computer. All the guard sees is a display that reads "MATCH" or "REJECT."

Inside the booth, the agent turns and faces a TV camera, and says his name and reads several phrases from a placard on the wall for a voiceprint.[5] The computer seeks a match, while the security guard checks the agent's face against a photo on his monitor. If the agent passes both checks, the guard will ask him to place his palm on a panel in front of him, where an optical reader records his palmprint for the computer to check against the one in its memory.[6]

Meanwhile, the guard manning the control panel is visually checking the agent against information displayed on the screen. As well as his photograph, his height and weight are on display, and the guard makes a visual determination of how closely they match. Behind the agent, as he stands in front of the TV camera, is a ruler on the wall, to allow the guard to estimate his height. The floor has a weight sensor, producing a readout on the screen in front of the guard. It's not necessary to have the computer compare the weights, and it might even be a source of errors, as weight varies according to many circumstances. A heavy meal, or heavy clothing, will increase weight by a couple of pounds. A human guard can understand that in winter, people dress more heavily and allow for that. In an adequate security system, the guard would know the people personally, and would be able to recognize progressive weight loss resulting from being on a diet, for example.

A computer is best for comparing features that don't vary, such as fingerprints. Variable features can cause false readings. That's why, in our hypothetical system, the guard visually matches the subject's face against a photo on a screen. Computer facial matching has been done, but a computer would not be able to differentiate between certain conditions and discrepancies that a human would recognize and discount immediately. A human guard will recognize the same person, even if he's growing a mustache, or has changed from eyeglasses to contact lenses.

Our hypothetical system is redundant. Only if the impostor passes all of the checks does the guard push the button that opens the inner door. If he fails, the outer door will open and the agent will find a couple of security guards waiting to escort him to the security office, where he'll undergo a further checkout.

In practice, electronic equipment sometimes fails, resulting in spurious readings. In our system, the agent has to pass several hurdles, and the system is designed against inadvertently passing an impostor. The expectation is that, even if one system fails, by equipment defect or by clever imposture by a penetrator, the others will detect discrepancies. This gives a greater chance of false rejection, but because of the importance of the high security area and the information contained within, the system's designers consider this to be an acceptable characteristic and the employers understand the need for it.

Electronic equipment isn't a substitute for intelligent and alert security guards, but an automated aid to speeding the process of personal identity verification. A human guard still has to make the final judgment.

If our agent passes all of the checks inside the booth, the door opens and he enters the high security area. Although the chances of his beating the security system are minuscule, we'll assume that he's done it to bring out a final point.

Inside, he'll come face to face with the subject's fellow employees, and will have to pass their scrutiny, casual though it may be. It's not enough to be a perfect physical match for the subject. The agent must also know the thousand details of the subject's job and the subtle interpersonal factors that go into it. If someone approaches and gives him an order, he must know whether or not that person is his supervisor, or someone merely making a power play. Another might approach him and ask, "Hey Jerry, are you coming to the big thing tonight?" To provide an appropriate answer, the agent must know what this "thing" is. If it's a party, he might beg off, but if he declines to attend a compulsory company meeting he'll cause himself complications.

Another may ask him, "Have you got that report for me?" The agent must know what the report is, and whether or not the subject has delayed it, to avoid giving an answer that may ring false.

The possibilities are endless. A fellow employee may tell him, "Phil's back." This is a simple declarative sentence, but it says little. The subject may know that Phil had been absent from work because his daughter had died, and would offer Phil his sympathy. An impersonator is unlikely to know the details of his fellow employees' lives, and would stumble over such points.

From the foregoing, we can see that, although making up to resemble another is possible if the physical match is close, a successful impersonation under close scrutiny is impossible. The impersonator would have to mimic too many characteristics, and would require too much specific knowledge, for him to carry it out. He would even have to learn to think like his subject. Even with modern methods of psychological conditioning, this is still science fiction, not fact.

Notes

1. Corson, Richard, *Stage Make-up*, 6th. Edition, Englewood Cliffs, NJ, Prentice-Hall, Inc., pp. 252-262.
2. Harrison G. Allison, *Personal Identification*, Boston, Holbrook Press, 1975, p. 5.
3. John Buchan, *The Thirty-Nine Steps,* NY, Popular Library, 1915.
4. Warfel, George H., *Identification Technologies*, Springfield, IL, Charles C. Thomas, Publisher, 1979, Chapter 7.
5. *Ibid.*, Chapter 6.
6. *Ibid.*, Chapter 5.

Appendix IV:

SOURCES FOR SUPPLIES AND SERVICES

Badges and I. D. Cards

Blackinton
221 John L. Dietsch Blvd.
PO Box 1300
Attleboro Falls, MA 02763-0300
Phone: (508) 699-4436
Fax: (508) 695-5349
    Blackinton is a police badge supply company.

Johnson Smith Company
4514 19th Street Court East
PO Box 25500
Bradenton, FL 34206-5500
Phone: (813) 747-2356

Fax: (813) 746-7896

Johnson Smith Company sells police-type and private investigator badges via mail-order, no questions asked.

NIC, Inc., Law Enforcement Supply
220 Carroll Street, Suite D
PO Box 5950
Shreveport, LA 71135-5950
Phone: (318) 222-2970
Fax: (318) 869-3228

NIC puts out a 112 page catalog listing badges, I.D. documents and cards, some of which are well-made replicas, and others genuine fakes, made to look like official documents but with non-existent titles. Examples are "Official Taxpayer," "Bail Enforcement Agent," "Registered Mercenary," and "Investigative Reporter." The catalog also lists books on conspiratorial topics, revenge, booby-traps, etc.

Roberts Company
180 Franklin Street
Framingham, MA 01701-6699
Phone: (800) 466-2677 for orders.
(508) 875-5852

The Badge Company
PO Box 5787
Parsippany, NJ 07054
Phone: (201) 263-9333

Camouflage Clothing

SHOMER-TEC
PO Box 2039
Bellingham, WA 98227

Phone: (206) 733-6214
Fax: (206) 676-5248

SHOMER-TEC also sells badges, police uniforms, and an array of police and para-military equipment. The catalog lists surveillance and tactical gear, and books on allied topics.

Casting Resin

Jonas Supply Co.
2260 Industrial Lane
Broomfield, CO 80020
Phone: (800) 525-6379 — Order desk only.
(303) 666-0101 — Other information.
Fax: (303) 666-9045

Contact Lenses

Ideal Optics
4000 Cumberland Parkway
Atlanta, GA 30339
Phone: (800) 554-7353
Fax: (414) 434-8291

Ideal Optics carries "Ciba Illusion" soft contact lenses, in various colors, which will change eye color. However, all contact lens orders have to go through an optometrist.

International Contact Lens Laboratory
63-52 Saunders Street
Rego Park, NY 11374
Phone: (800) 422-8489

International provides contact lenses to change eye color, but they must be ordered through an optometrist.

Costumes, Uniforms, and Work Clothes

Badger Uniform Company
1125 Sixth Street
Racine, WI 53401
Phone: (800) 558-5952

Broadway Costumes, Inc.
954 West Washington Blvd.
Fourth Floor
Chicago, IL 60607
Phone: (800) 397-3316 or (312) 829-6400
Fax: (312) 829-8621

Broadway Costumes is an outlet for both costumes and make-up. The cosmetic line includes Ben Nye, Bob Kelly, Kryolan, and Stein. Beards and mustaches are also available.

The costume line is for rental only, and includes uniforms for bands, bell hops, bus drivers, delivery services, doorman, firemen, house painters, medical personnel, police officers, postal carriers, security guards, ushers, waiters, etc. A limited array of contemporary military uniforms is also in the line.

Creative Costumes Co.
Sales & Rentals
330 West 38th Street
New York, NY
Phone: (212) 564-5552

Some's Uniforms, Inc.
65 Route 17
Paramus, NJ 07652-0306
Phone: (201) 843-1199

Some's provides a 304 page catalog listing uniforms, patches, and accessories for a variety of occupations, such as police officer, security guard, firefighter, postal carrier, military, hotel and restaurant employees, and transportation personnel. This is available for $50 for individuals, but free to police when requested on a department letterhead.

Special Duty
2855 Centennial Avenue
Radcliff, KY 40160-9000
Phone: (800) 777-7732 or (800) 333-5102 or (502) 351-1164
Fax: (502) 352-0266
   "Special Duty" puts out uniforms and S.W.A.T. gear made by U.S. Cavalry, as well as a variety of special gear such as gloves, gear bags, and other police and military related equipment.

I. Spiewak & Sons
505 Eighth Avenue
New York, NY 10018
Phone: (800) 223-6850
Fax: (212) 629-4803

Topps Mfg. Company
501 Main Street
PO Box 750
Rochester, IN 46975
Phone: (800) 348-2990 or (219) 223-4311
Fax: (219) 223-8622
   Topps supplies uniforms, specializing in jump suits, which are of high quality and moderately priced.

WearGuard Work Clothes
Longwater Drive
Norwell, MA 02061
Phone: (800) 388-3300

WearGuard sells a variety of uniforms, appropriate to delivery men and women, utility company employees, street workers, mechanics, health care workers, security personnel, and construction workers.

Also included are boots and work shoes, knit caps, baseball caps, and gloves. WearGuard will, on special order, screen print most garments with professional logos, including those appropriate to delivery services, fire departments, paramedics, aviation, construction, auto repair, and many others.

Make-up

Bob Kelly Cosmetics, Inc.
151 West 46th Street
New York, NY 10036
Phone: (212) 819-0030
Kelly carries a variety of make-up products made for use on stage, screen, and television. These include creme stick, eye liner and shadow, spirit gum and remover, cosmetic pencils, special effect waxes, brushes, latex, make-up kits, and wigs.

Broadway Costumes, Inc.
954 West Washington Blvd.
Fourth Floor
Chicago, IL 60607
Phone: (800) 397-3316 or (312) 829-6400
Fax: (312) 829-8621
Broadway Costumes is an outlet for both costumes and make-up. The cosmetic line includes Ben Nye, Bob Kelly, Kryolan, and Stein. Beards and mustaches are also available.

Cabot Laboratories
Central Islip, New York, 11722

Cabot makes "Clear Perfection." This line includes corrective cover creme, corrective finishing powder, corrective retouch concealer, and leg & body cover creme.

Jack Stein Make-up Center
186 South Street
Boston, MA 02111
Phone: (800) 562-3217 or (617) 542-7865
Jack Stein provides a variety of theatrical make-up products, including foundations, cremes, lipsticks, and even wigs.

Max Factor Cosmetics was recently purchased by:
Proctor & Gamble
PO Box 599
Cincinnati, OH 45201
Phone: (800) 283-4879.
Max Factor makes powders, cremes, concealer, lipstick, and a variety of theatrical make-up products.

Mehron, Inc.
45E Route 303
Valley Cottage, NY 10989
Phone: (800) 332-9955 or (914) 268-4106
Mehron supplies individual items, such as cake make-up, and kits. Some items, such as Texas Dirt Powder and stage blood, are unusual. Make-up kits include arrays of powders, cakes, sponges, brushes, etc., in several types: male, female, Black, and TV-video. A special type is clown make-up.

Nishimoto Trading Company
2747 S. Maly Avenue
Los Angeles, CA 90040
Phone: (800) 835-8844

Nishimoto supplies "Bigen," a powder hair coloring product that adheres when mixed with water. This is a surface coloring, not a hair dye.

Schering-Plough
Memphis, TN 38151
Schering-Plough makes "Coppertone."

Sig Frends Beauty Supply
5270 Laurel Canyon Blvd.
North Hollywood, CA 91607
Phone: (213) 877-4828 or (818) 769-3834
Sig Frends carries a variety of make-up supplies, including make-up removing creams, hair brushes, lip liner, make-up brushes, scar material, pancake make-up, spirit gum and removers, color foundations, molding wax, mold release, mustaches and beards, prosthetic adhesive, prosthetic paints, and other special effects materials.

Zauder Brothers., Inc.
10 Henry Street
Freeport, NY 11520
Phone: (516) 379-2600
Fax: (516) 223-3397
Zauder Bros. operates Stein's Theatrical Make-up, and the catalog lists many standard make-up items, as well as clown wigs and colors. One significant item is nose putty, for a quick and disposable nose augmentation job.

Prostheses

Glenn Reams, Ocularist (artificial eyes)
407 Park Street
Waterloo, IL 62298

Phone: (800) 426-8995

This supplier provides artificial eyes custom-made by doctor's order. Buyer has choice of stock or custom eyes. The material of choice today is plastic, not glass.

Mobility Orthopedics
2515 Fall Hill Avenue
Fredericksburg, VA 22401
Phone: (800) 247-5543

Mobility furnishes both orthodics (braces) and prostheses (replacement parts) upon order of a physician.

Quick & Dirty Disguises

Johnson Smith Company
4514 19th Street Court East
PO Box 25500
Bradenton, FL 34206-5500
Phone: (813) 747-2356
Fax: (813) 746-7896

Johnson Smith is a mail order supplier for "nerd" glasses, false mustaches, panoramic sunglasses with side shields, and mirror sunglasses. Smith also sells props, such as a fake cellular phone.

Shoe Lifts

Inner Lifts
PO Box 828
Apex, NC 27502
Phone: (919) 387-7766
Fax: (919) 362-0863
Attn: Ed Andrews

Richlee Shoe Company
PO Box 3566
Frederick, MD 21701
Phone: (800) 343-3810 or (301) 663-5111
NOTE: Richlee also does business under the name of "Elevators."

Silicon Rubber

Circle K Products
20814 S. Normandie Avenue
Torrance, CA 90502
Phone: (714) 695-1955
Fax: (714) 695-0605

R. H. Carlson Company
510 Maltbie Street
Lawrenceville, GA 30205
Phone: (800) 241-9006 or (404) 962-4461
Fax: (404) 962-0823

Hastings Plastics
1704 Colorado Avenue
Santa Monica, CA 90404
Phone: (310) 829-3449
Fax: (310) 828-6820

GE Silicones
Silicone Customer Development
260 Hudson River Road
Waterford, NY 12188
Phone: (800) 255-8886 or (518) 233-3330

Silicones, Inc.
PO Box 363
High Point, NC 27261
Phone: (919) 886-5018
Fax: (919) 886-7122

Wacker Silicones
Phone: (800) 248-0061
This toll-free number is for customer service, which will provide the toll-free number of the nearest regional office.
California: (800) 541-9517

Skin Tanning Preparations

Bain de Soleil
Proctor & Gamble
PO Box 599
Cincinnati, OH 45201
Phone: (800) 283-4879.

Tattoos

Arrow Specialties
1810 Louis Lane
Hastings, MN 55033
Phone: (612) 437-9671
Arrow sells removable tattoos made on poly film which when wet, adhere to the skin. These last for several days, and don't wash off in water, although removable with soap.

Don Ling's Removable Tattoos and Fantoos
PO Box 309
Butterfield, MN 56120
Phone: (800) 247-6817 or (507) 956-2024

Fax: (507) 956-2060

This company sells temporary tattoos, applied with water and removable with baby oil, which last for several days. Don Ling supplies a sample tattoo with his brochure.

Tooth Whitener

EPI Products
PO Box 2975
Beverly Hills, CA 90213
Phone: (800) 444-5347

Transvestite Publications and Supplies

Sources of apparel and other items for cross-dressing are:

E.H.B. (Also operates under name of "Especially For Me")
PO Box 1489
Ontario, CA 91862
Phone: (714) 946-6251
Fax: (714) 946-5500

E.H.B. carries breast items, rubber pants, slips and other underwear, gloves, wigs, breast forms, and other TV items. Also publishes a catalog.

Laura Lee
PO Box 711
Farmingdale, NJ 07727-0711

Laura Lee advertises in various tabloids.

Versatile Fashions
PO Box 1051
Tustin, CA 92681
Phone: (714) 538-6498

Versatile Fashion's boutique is located at:
1925 E. Lincoln Avenue
Anaheim, CA 92805
Phone: (714) 776-1510

Publications and other media materials relating to transvestitism are available from:

Classic Publications
PO Box 2113
Apple Valley, CA 92307

Classic sells erotic stories covering bondage and restraint.

Ground Zero Enterprises, Ltd.
PO Box 7575
LaVerne, CA 91750

Publishes *TV Sexcapades*, a tabloid for transvestites that includes personal ads, phone hot lines, and sources of materials and supplies.

Letro Limited
PO Box 2966
Mission Viejo, CA 92690

Letro Limited sells "adult" videos, covering the following topics: Hermaphrodites, She-Male, TV, Pregnant, Amateur, B&D, and other hard to find videos.

Tania Volen
PO Box 280
Tennent, NJ 07763-0280

Tania Volen publishes *Dateline, Discipline, Femanine, Leather and Lace, Players, The Sophisticate, TransForm,* and *The Transvestian.*

Vitamin-A Creme

Prescription-only "Retin-A" is manufactured by Ortho Pharmaceuticals, and is available through local pharmacies.

Non-prescription "Retinol" is available via mail-order from:

Beauty Solutions
334 East Lake Rd., Suite 171
Palm Harbor, FL 34685

Voice Changing Devices

Eavesdropping Detection Equipment
PO Box 337
Buffalo, NY 14226
Phone: (716) 691-3476
Fax: (716) 691-0604
E.D.E. provides a digital, battery-powered voice changer that goes over the phone's mouthpiece, and includes a button-activated barking dog simulator.

Operative Supply
PO Box 2343
Atlantic Beach, NC 28512
Phone: (919) 726-1582
Operative Supply provides three models of electronic voice changers. One is a small digital voice changer powered by one 9-volt battery. Another, powered by four AA batteries, installs between handset and phone on two-piece telephones, and provides 16 voice changing levels. The third is a telephone with built-in voice changer.

Productive Electronic Products
PO Box 930024
Norcross, GA 30093
Phone: (404) 938-0381

    P.E.P. makes the "vocomask," a battery-powered device that goes between the handset and body of a two-piece telephone, and digitally changes the voice's pitch.

Wigs and Hairpieces

Afro World
7276 Natural Bridge
St. Louis, MO 63121
Phone: (800) 325-8067 or (314) 389-5194
Fax: (314) 389-8508

    Afro World specializes in ethnic wigs, including Black, Caucasian, Latin, and Asian, using 100% human hair. Male and female hairpieces available.

Beauty by Spector, Inc.
Dept. MOD-93
McKeesport, PA 15134-0502
Phone: (412) 673-3529
Attn: Myer Spector, Pres.

    Beauty by Spector provides hairgoods for both men and women. These are custom, not stock, hairpieces, and are made to order. These are made of synthetic fibers, and Spector strongly recommends you send a sample of your hair, such as from a recent haircut, for an accurate color match.

Beauty Trends
PO Box 9323
Hialeah, FL 33014-9323
Phone: (800) 777-7772 or (305) 826-8283

Beauty Trends provides budget-priced female wigs, starting at $29. The catalog recommends sending a hair sample for closest match. The catalog also contains color charts for both the Revlon and Adolfo wig lines.

Carla Corsini
PO Box 1700
Brockton, MA 02403-1700
Phone: (800) 229-1234

Carla Corsini supplies synthetic hair wigs. The catalog lists dozens of full and partial wig styles, with color charts for matching. The catalog recommends sending a pencil-thick swatch of hair at least 1" long for best color matching.

Bob Ellis
280 Driggs Avenue
Brooklyn, NY 11222
Phone: (718) 383-3779

Ellis recommends that you send a swatch of your hair for close matching. Offers both natural and synthetic hairpieces.

Franklin Fashions Corp.
103 E. Hawthorne Avenue
Valley Stream, NY 11582
Phone: (800) 556-0034 or (516) 561-6260
Fax: (516) 568-0259

Franklin makes both male and female wigs, including a "Black is beautiful" collection.

King Hairpieces for Men
2730 Octavia
San Francisco, CA 94123
Phone: (415) 771-3392

Recommends sending a hair sample for matching.

Nina-America
40 West 27th Street, 11th Floor
New York, NY 10001
Phone: (800) 292-6462 or (212) 683-6462
Fax:(212) 683-6646

Nina-America provides both human hair and synthetic female wigs in a variety of colors and styles suitable for several ethnic types.

Paula Young
Phone: (800) 472-4017
Will send catalog.

Top-Man
35 Java Street
San Francisco, CA 94117
Phone: (415) 454-6224

Top-Man supplies synthetic hairpieces for men, as well as medical quality hairpiece tape, Vapon no-tape adhesive liquid, and Chromatone spray hair color restorer. Suggests sending a hair sample for accurate matching.

The Wig Company
Box 12950
Pittsburgh, PA 15241
Phone: (800) 245-6288 or (800) 444-1788 or (800) 456-1788 or (412) 221-4794
Fax: (412) 257-8181

The Wig Company specializes in female wigs in a variety of colors and styles. The catalog suggests choosing a color from the printed selection guide, or sending a sample of your own hair for matching. The Wig Company will even send a wig fiber swatch to let the customer see it before making the final decision.

Wigs by Genie
Phone: (800) 922-9447
Will send brochure.

Yellow Pages

The classified directory is a good guide to local sources. Categories to cover are; cosmetics, hair, hair products, make-up, prostheses, stage and theatrical make-up, and wigs.

Appendix V:

FOR FURTHER READING

Decircumcision, Gary Griffin, Los Angeles, CA, Added Dimensions Publishing, 1991. Griffin's 108-page softcover book is a short, practical workbook on foreskin restoration. It covers both surgical and non-surgical methods, with illustrations complementing the text.

Disguise Techniques, Edmond A. MacInaugh, Boulder, CO, Paladin Press, 1984. This 82-page softcover book contains six chapters providing an overview of the philosophy of disguise, and covering specific techniques. The author rightly points out that attitude and mannerisms, including gait, contribute greatly to the success of the effort.

Foreskin Restoration, By Mark Waring, Metairie, LA, Privately printed, 1988. This 64-page softcover book is the first book dealing with foreskin restoration, detailing both surgical and non-surgical methods. It deals briefly with the history of foreskin restoration from Greco-Roman times, through the efforts of Jews to restore their foreskins during the Nazi era, and covers modern times when many circumcised males have formed support groups and other organizations to pursue non-surgical restoration. The author's credentials are impressive, as he underwent non-surgical restoration himself, and obtained most of his information first-hand and from others with first-hand experience in the various surgical and non-surgical methods. Unfortunately, some of the information is now out of date, and there have been new developments since this book's publication. This book is out of print, and no second edition ever appeared.

Guide To Cosmetic Surgery, Josleen Wilson, New York, Simon & Schuster, 1992. This book, produced under the auspices of the American Society of Plastic and Reconstructive Surgeons, is the "official" text on the subject. As such, it provides a good, step-by-step blueprint on topics such as finding a plastic surgeon, and good descriptions of the most commonly performed operations, such as facelifts and tummy tucks. It does not discuss areas that don't have official recognition, such as fingerprint suppression, foreskin restoration, and sex-change surgery. We do find interesting and important points in this book, and readers should pay close attention to them. One is that plastic surgeons expect you to pay them "without regard to the outcome" (Page 67) and that they want their fees in advance (Pages 67 and 68). Also important are the lists of problems and complications that can follow any plastic surgery operation. If you're considering any sort of plastic surgery, read these parts and take them seriously!

Identification Technologies, George H. Warfel, Springfield, IL, Charles C. Thomas, Publisher, 1979. At the time of writing, this book described cutting edge technologies for personal identification. Some of the techniques described are in common use today, while others are just coming into service in limited ways. This book is a comprehensive reference work on what's possible and what's not in the field of personal identification.

The Joy Of Uncircumcising!, by Jim Bigelow, Ph. D., Aptos, CA, Hourglass Publishing, 1992. This 240 page book is the most recent, and the most comprehensive, description of foreskin restoration techniques from past to present. This thoroughly researched volume examines all known methods of foreskin restoration to date, and their variations. It contains many drawings and photographs to illustrate the discussions, and provides careful appraisals of the advantages and disadvantages of each class of restoration technique. At the time of writing, this is by far the best book on the topic.

The Prop Builder's Mask-Making Handbook, by Thurston James, available from Hastings Plastics.

Stage Make-Up, 6th Edition, Richard Corson, Englewood Cliffs, NJ, Prentice-Hall, Inc. This is a basic American text on stage and movie make-up by a practitioner in the field.

The Technique Of The Professional Make-Up Artist, Vincent J-R Kehoe, Boston, Focal Press, 1985. This book focuses on make-up in context with TV, film, or the stage. The discussion of light and its effects on make-up is interesting reading, because it shows how make-up made for one situation can be inadequate in another. The rest of the book is a methodical discussion, illustrated by many photographs, of each make-up technique. Some, such as monster make-up, won't be very useful for disguise, but conservative applications of the techniques shown will change facial features and contours.

Theatrical Make-Up, Bert Broe, London, Pelham Books, 1984. This book contains an exceptional number of color and black-and-white photographs illustrating the step-by-step instructions. The text covers many make-up effects, including aging and others.

Three-Dimensional Make-Up, Lee Baygan, New York, Watson-Guptill Publications, 1982. The author concentrates on what he calls "prosthetic" make-up, going beyond grease pencil and face powder. He explains and demonstrates using molded pieces of foam, latex, and other materials to change facial contours and features, using hundreds of black & white and color photographs to illustrate every step.

One chapter describes modifying the teeth, using acrylics to produce outlandish effects such as vampire teeth. Another deals with changing the shape of the ears with latex add-ons. Thus, small, flat ears can be changed to prominent jug ears, strongly modifying appearance.

YOU WILL ALSO WANT TO READ:

☐ **61115 REBORN IN THE U.S.A., Personal Privacy Through a New Identity, Second Edition,** *by Trent Sands.* A complete guide to building a new identity in the United States from the ground up. Covers birth certificates, Social Security cards, drivers licenses, passports, credit cards, and much more. Learn how to thoroughly document your new identity without revealing any information about your former life. *1991, 5½ x 8½, 121 pp, soft cover.* **$14.95.**

☐ **61131 REBORN WITH CREDIT,** *by Trent Sands.* Trent Sands takes you inside the credit machine to show you how credit applications are processed and graded, how credit bureaus get their information, and how credit decisions are made. The master of identity then takes you step-by-step through procedures for cleaning bad credit, establishing a blank credit file, and building a credit rating that will make tens of thousands of dollars available to you in a matter of months. *1992, 5½ x 8½, 72 pp, soft cover.* **$10.00.**

☐ **61129 UNDERSTANDING U.S. IDENTITY DOCUMENTS,** *by John Q. Newman.* The most detailed examination of identity documents ever published. Covers birth certificates, Social Security cards, drivers licenses and passports. It shows how each document is generated and used, and explains the strengths and weaknesses of the agencies issuing them. An essential reference for anyone concerned with their official identity and how it is maintained and manipulated. *1991, 8½ x 11, 207 pp, illustrated, soft cover.* **$25.00.**

☐ **61138 SCRAM: Relocating Under A New Identity,** *by James S. Martin.* This new book includes ten real-life case histories that show the problems and opportunities for identity-changes, along with a question/answer format. Chapters include: The Commitment to a new identity, Personal reorganization, New identity papers, Tracing missing persons, Changing your looks, Police searches, The right to travel, Faking death, Chances for success. If you have ever wondered what it would be like to start over, check out *SCRAM! 1993, 5½ x 8½, 83 pp, soft cover.* **$12.00.**

LOOMPANICS UNLIMITED   **MOD29**
PO BOX 1197
PORT TOWNSEND, WA 98368

Please send me the titles I have checked above. I have enclosed $_____ which includes $4.00 for the shipping and handling of 1 to 3 books, $6.00 for 4 or more.

Name _____

Address_____

City _____

State/Zip _____

(Washington residents please include 7.8% sales tax.)

THE BEST BOOK CATALOG IN THE WORLD!!!

We offer hard-to-find books on the world's most unusual subjects. Here are a few of the topics covered IN DEPTH in our exciting new catalog:

- *Hiding/Concealment of physical objects! A complete section of the best books ever written on hiding things.*
- *Fake ID/Alternate Identities! The most comprehensive selection of books on this little-known subject ever offered for sale! You have to see it to believe it!*
- *Investigative/Undercover methods and techniques! Professional secrets known only to a few, now revealed to you to use! Actual police manuals on shadowing and surveillance!*
- *And much, much more, including Locks and Lockpicking, Self-Defense, Intelligence Increase, Life Extension, Money-Making Opportunities, Human Oddities, Exotic Weapons, Sex, Drugs, Anarchism, and more!*

Our book catalog is 280 pages, 8½ x 11, packed with over 800 of the most controversial and unusual books ever printed! You can order every book listed! Periodic supplements keep you posted on the LATEST titles available!!! Our catalog is $5.00, including shipping and handling.

Our book catalog is truly THE BEST BOOK CATALOG IN THE WORLD! Order yours today. You will be very pleased, we know.

LOOMPANICS UNLIMITED
PO BOX 1197
PORT TOWNSEND, WA 98368
USA